The Parent's Success Guide™ to Baby Planning

Edited by P. Weverka

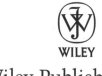

WILEY

Wiley Publishing, Inc.

The Parent's Success Guide™ to Baby Planning

Published by
Wiley Publishing, Inc.
111 River St.
Hoboken, NJ 07030-5774
www.wiley.com

For general information on our other products and services or to obtain technical support, please contact our Customer Care Department within the U.S. at 800-762-2974, outside the U.S. at 317-572-3993, or fax 317-572-4002.

Wiley also publishes its books in a variety of electronic formats. Some content that appears in print may not be available in electronic books.

Library of Congress Control Number: 2003114880

ISBN: 0-7645-5925-7

Manufactured in the United States of America

10 9 8 7 6 5 4 3 2 1

1V/SS/RS/QT/IN

WILEY

About the Authors

Keith Eddleman, MD, works at The Mount Sinai Medical Center. He is also a full-time faculty member in the Division of Maternal-Fetal Medicine, director of Prenatal Diagnosis, and coauthor of *Pregnancy For Dummies.*

Mary Murray, a former newspaper reporter, has been a magazine writer and editor since the mid-1980s. She is a coauthor of *Pregnancy For Dummies.*

Joanne Stone, MD, is a full-time faculty member in the Division of Maternal-Fetal Medicine at The Mount Sinai Medical Center in New York. She is the director of the Perinatal Ultrasound Unit, cares for patients with problem pregnancies, and coauthored *Pregnancy For Dummies.*

Marlene Targ Brill is an author, early childhood specialist, and special educator. She holds a master's degree in early childhood education from Roosevelt University. She authored *Raising Smart Kids For Dummies,* among many other books.

Dan Gookin is the author of many *For Dummies* computer books, including the first ever, *DOS For Dummies.* He coauthored *Parenting For Dummies,* 2nd Edition.

Sandra Hardin Gookin holds a BA degree in speech communications from Oklahoma State University. She is the mother of four boys and coauthor of *Parenting For Dummies,* 2nd Edition.

Peter Weverka is the author of several *For Dummies* computer books and also a coauthor of books in the health field. He edited this book.

Publisher's Acknowledgements

Some of the people who helped bring this book to market include the following:

Editor: Tere Drenth

Acquisitions Editors: Holly Gastineau-Grimes, Joyce Pepple

Technical Reviewer: Denise Meeks, RN, CNM, MSN

Cover Photo: © Getty Images

Illustrator: Kathryn Born

Table of Contents

Table of Contents

Part 3: What You've Been Waiting For: The Big Day 73

Chapter 7: Labor Day – More Than a Sign to Stop Wearing White...75

Chapter 8: Thirty Minutes or Less? Doubtful! The Delivery 91

Table of Contents

Part 1
A Little Bit Pregnant

If your first thought when you discover you're pregnant is, "I'm not sure I'm ready for this," you're having a completely normal reaction, no matter how much thought you've put into having a baby. Suddenly, you're faced with the fact that your body is changing and a baby is taking shape inside you. And although you may not feel ready, preparing for the 40 weeks ahead is easy enough. This part explains the many ways you can plan ahead for the very important and very interesting months ahead of you.

Chapter 1

Before You Try and Finding Out You Succeeded

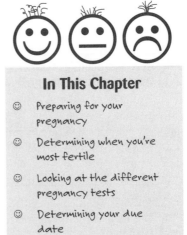

In This Chapter

☺ Preparing for your pregnancy

☺ Determining when you're most fertile

☺ Looking at the different pregnancy tests

☺ Determining your due date

Congratulations! If you're already pregnant, you're about to embark on one of the most exciting adventures of your life. The next year will be filled with tremendous changes and, with any luck, unbelievable happiness. And if you're thinking about getting pregnant but aren't pregnant yet, you're probably excited at the prospect but also a little nervous, too.

This chapter describes how to get your body ready for your pregnancy and also offers advice for conceiving. You uncover various methods of testing for pregnancy and discover the signals your body sends when you're pregnant. Of course, you want to know when your baby is due, so this chapter also tells you how to calculate your due date and explains why pregnancy is actually 40 weeks, not nine months.

First Things First: Using This Book

This book is part of a series called *The Parent's Success Guide*. Its main purpose is to help you, a busy, multitasking mom (or dad!), make some positive changes in your life as a parent — in a minimum amount of time.

Brought to you by the makers of the world-famous *For Dummies* series, this book provides straightforward advice, hands-on information, and helpful, practical tips — all of it on, about, and for being a smart parent. And this book does so with warmth, encouragement, and gentleness — as a trusted friend would do.

This book isn't meant to be read from front to back, so you don't have to read the entire book to understand what's going on. Just go to the chapter or section that interests you. Keep an eye out for text in italics, which indicates a new term and a nearby definition — no need to spend time hunting through a glossary.

While reading this book, you'll see these icons sprinkled here and there:

 This icon points out advice that saves time, requires less effort, achieves a quick result, or helps make a task easier.

 This icon signifies information that's important to keep in mind.

 This icon alerts you to areas of caution or danger — negative information you need to be aware of.

The Parent's Success Guide to Baby Planning is the happy offspring of three *For Dummies* books. If you'd like more comprehensive information about a particular subject covered in this book, you may want to pick up a copy of the *For Dummies* book covering the same topic. This book consists primarily of text compiled from

❋ *Pregnancy For Dummies*

❋ *Parenting For Dummies, 2nd Edition*

❋ *Raising Smart Kids For Dummies*

The Easiest Way to Get Pregnant

This book assumes that you know the basics of how to get pregnant! What you may not know, however, is how to make the process efficient so that you give yourself the best chance of getting pregnant. To do that, you need to think about *ovulation*, or the releasing of an egg from your ovary. Ovulation occurs once each cycle (usually once per month).

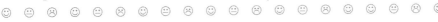
After leaving the ovary, the egg spends a couple of days gliding down the fallopian tube, until it reaches the uterus (also know as the womb), as shown in Figure 1-1. Most often pregnancy occurs when the egg is fertilized within 24 hours of its release from the ovary, during its passage through the tube, and the budding embryo then implants into the lining of the uterus. In order to get pregnant, your job (yours and the father-to-be's) is to get the sperm to meet up with the egg as soon as possible. Ideally, the sperm and egg meet within 12 to 24 hours of ovulation.

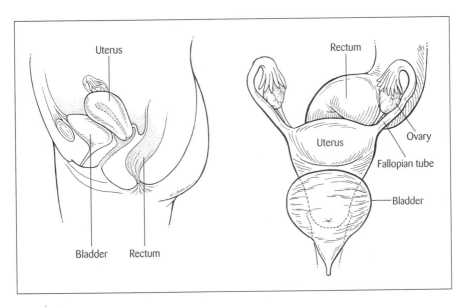

Figure 1-1: The female productive system.

Typically, ovulation happens about 14 days before you get your period. If you have a 28-day menstrual cycle, ovulation occurs about 14 days after the first day of your previous period. If you have a 32-day cycle, you probably ovulate about 18 days after your previous period. To make sure you get the sperm in the right place at the right time, have sex several times around the time of ovulation, starting five days before you expect to ovulate and continuing for two or three days afterward.

 The absolute prime time to have sex is 12 hours prior to ovulation, because then the sperm are in place as soon as the egg comes out. Sperm are thought to live inside a woman's body for only 24 to 48 hours, although some have been known to fertilize eggs when they are as much as seven days old.

Quitting birth control

How soon can you get pregnant after you stop using birth control? That depends. Whereas the barrier methods — condoms, diaphragms, and spermicides — work only as long as you use them, hormone-based medicines — the Pill, Depo-Provera, and Norplant — take longer to get out of your system. You may ovulate very shortly after stopping the Pill, but you may need three months to a year to resume regular ovulatory cycles after stopping Depo-Provera.

Keep in mind that if you haven't resumed regular cycles, you may not be ovulating each month, so you may have more difficulty timing your intercourse to achieve conception. At least you can have a good time trying!

No couple should count on getting pregnant on the first try. On average, you have a 15 to 25 percent chance each month. Studies have shown that roughly half of all couples trying to get pregnant conceive within four months. By six months, three-fourths of them make it; by a year, 85 percent do; and by two years the success rate is up to 93 percent. If you have been trying unsuccessfully to conceive for a year or more, a fertility evaluation is warranted.

"I Think I'm Pregnant"

Quite often, the first sign of being pregnant is a missed period, but your body gives off many other signals, sometimes even sooner than that first missed period, and these signals typically grow more noticeable with each passing week. Some women experience one or two days of light bleeding. This is known as *implantation bleeding* because the embryo is attaching itself to the lining of the uterus.

You may become ravenous for pickles, pasta, and other particular foods, yet turn up your nose at things you normally love to eat. What you've heard about a pregnant woman's appetite is true. Experts suspect that these changes are, at least partly, nature's way of ensuring that you get the proper nutrients. You may also be very thirsty early in pregnancy. The extra water you drink is useful for increasing your body's supply of blood and other fluids.

You'll be amazed at how early in pregnancy your breasts begin to grow. In fact, large and tender breasts are often the first symptom of pregnancy that you feel. Early in pregnancy, levels of estrogen and progesterone rise, causing immediate changes in your breasts.

☺ ☺ ☹ ☺ ☺ ☹ ☺ ☺ ☹ ☺ ☺ ☹ ☺ ☺ ☹ ☺ ☺ ☺ ☺ ☹ ☺

Testing, Testing, 1, 2, 3

These days, you don't need to go to your practitioner's office (see Chapter 2) to find out whether you're pregnant. Here are the different pregnancy tests you can take:

✱ **Home test (urine test):** The tests you can purchase at a drugstore are basically simplified chemistry sets, designed to check for the presence in your urine of human chorionic gonadotropin, or hCG, the hormone produced by the developing placenta. These kits are not as precise as laboratory tests that look for hCG in blood, but they can provide positive results very quickly — by the day you miss your period, or about two weeks after conception.

Even if you had a positive home pregnancy test, most practitioners want to confirm this test in their office before beginning the rest of your prenatal care. Your practitioner may decide to simply repeat a urine pregnancy test or to use a blood pregnancy test, instead.

✱ **Blood test:** A blood pregnancy test checks for hCG in your blood. This test can be either qualitative (a simple positive or negative result) or quantitative (an actual measurement of the amount of hCG in your blood). The test your practitioner chooses depends in part upon your history and your current symptoms, and in part on his or her individual preference. A blood test, which is the more accurate of the two, can be positive even when urine tests are negative.

Calculating Your Due Date

Pinpointing your due date as precisely as possible is important in order to ensure that the tests you need along the way are performed at the right time. Knowing how far along you are also makes it easier for your doctor to see that the baby is growing properly. (By the way, only 1 in 20 women delivers on her due date. Most women deliver anywhere from three weeks early to two weeks late.)

If your menstrual cycles are 28 days long, you can use the following worksheet to pinpoint your due date:

_____ Date your last period started

− _____ Less three months

+ _____ Plus 7 days

= _____ Due date

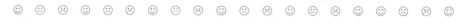

Weeks versus months

Most people think of pregnancy as lasting nine months. But face it: Forty weeks is a little longer than nine times four weeks. It's closer to ten lunar months (in Japan, they actually speak of pregnancy as lasting ten months) and a bit longer than nine 30-to-31-day calendar months. That's why your doctor is more likely to talk in terms of weeks.

Because you start counting from the date of your last menstrual period (LMP), you actually start the count a couple of weeks *before* you conceive. So when your doctor says you're 12 weeks pregnant, the fetus is really only 10 weeks old!

The average pregnancy lasts 280 days, or 40 weeks, counting from the first day of the last menstrual period. To calculate your due date, begin with the date on which your last menstrual period (LMP) started. If your cycles are 28 days long, you can calculate your due date by subtracting three months from your LMP and adding seven days. If your last period started on June 3, for example, your due date would be March (subtract three months) 10 (add seven days).

 If your periods didn't follow 28-day cycles, don't worry. You can establish your due date in other ways. If you can pinpoint the date of conception, coming up with an accurate date is especially easy. If not, you can get an ultrasound exam during the first three months to get a good idea of your due date. A first trimester ultrasound predicts your due date more accurately than a second or third trimester one.

To tell how far along you are at any given moment, you can either keep track of the number of days that have passed since your last period or use a pregnancy wheel. You can usually obtain one at your practitioner's office or at a birth resource centers. To use this handy tool, line up the arrow to the date of your last menstrual period and then look for today's date. Just below the date you see the number of weeks and days that have gone by. You can see what a pregnancy wheel looks like in Figure 1-2.

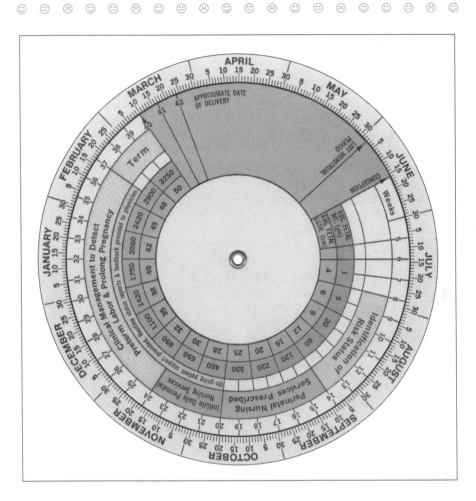

Figure 1-2: A sample pregnancy wheel.

Part 1: A Little Bit Pregnant

☺ ☺ ☹ ☺ ☺ ☹ ☺ ☺ ☹ ☺ ☺ ☹ ☺ ☺ ☹ ☺ ☺ ☺ ☹ ☺

Chapter 2

Preparing for the Next Nine Months

When pregnant, your body undergoes miraculous changes, but your day-to-day life somehow still has to go on. You have a lot to consider, from choosing a practitioner to figuring how much your life needs to change, now that you're pregnant. This chapter discusses some of the lifestyle changes you can expect throughout your pregnancy, including what to expect at your first prenatal visit. See Chapter 3 for two additional lifestyle changes: eating and exercising.

Choosing a Practitioner Who's Right for You

After you finish celebrating the results of your positive pregnancy test, you need to get down to business and think about what lies ahead. The next step is to decide who your practitioner is and give the office a call.

Midwives, obstetricians, maternal-fetal specialists — many kinds of professionals can help you through pregnancy and delivery. Be sure to choose a practitioner with whom you feel comfortable. Here is a list of the basic four:

❁ **Obstetrician/gynecologist (ob/gyn):** This physician has four years of special training in pregnancy, delivery, and women's health. He or she should be *board certified* (or be in the process of becoming board certified) by the American Board of Obstetrics and Gynecology or an equivalent program if you're from a country other than the United States.

❁ **Maternal-fetal medicine specialist (also known as a *perinatologist* or *high-risk obstetrician*):** This type of doctor has completed a two-to-three-year fellowship in the care of high-risk

☺ ☺ ☹ ☺ ☺ ☹ ☺ ☺ ☹ ☺ ☺ ☹ ☺ ☺ ☹ ☺ ☺ ☹ ☺

pregnancies, on top of the standard obstetrics residency, to become board certified in maternal-fetal medicine.

❀ **Family practice physician:** This doctor provides general medical care for whole families — men, women, and children. He or she is board certified in family practice medicine. This kind of doctor is likely to refer you to an obstetrician or maternal-fetal medicine specialist if complications arise during your pregnancy.

❀ **Certified nurse-midwife:** A certified nurse-midwife is a registered nurse who is certified in the care of pregnant women and is also licensed to perform deliveries. A certified nurse-midwife often practices in conjunction with a physician and refers patients to a specialist when complications occur.

How soon your first visit will be scheduled depends in part on your past and current health history. If you haven't been on prenatal vitamins or other folic-acid-containing vitamins, let the office know. Someone at the office will be able to call in a prescription for prenatal vitamins so that you can start taking them even before your first prenatal visit.

Prenatal Visits

Your practitioner does some things consistently from trimester to trimester — like checking your blood pressure, urine, and the baby's heartbeat, and those checkups are discussed in this chapter. (Chapters 4, 5, and 6 go over the specifics of what happens during prenatal visits in each trimester.) Table 2-1 gives you an overview of the typical schedule for prenatal visits and what happens at each visit.

Table 2-1 Prenatal Visits

Stage of Pregnancy	Frequency of Doctor Visits
First visit to 28 weeks	Every four weeks
28 to 36 weeks	Every two to three weeks
36 weeks to delivery	Weekly

Prenatal visits vary a bit according to each woman's personal needs and each practitioner's style. Some women need particular laboratory tests or physical examinations. But a few measures and checks are standard during each prenatal visit:

❀ **A nurse checks your weight and blood pressure.** For more information on how much weight you should be gaining and when, see Chapter 3.

❀ **You give a urine sample (usually an easy job for most pregnant women!).** Your practitioner checks for the presence of protein or glucose to look for any signs of preeclampsia (see Chapter 6) or diabetes (discussed in Chapter 5).

❀ **A nurse or doctor listens for and counts the baby's heartbeat.** Typically, the heartbeat ranges between 120 and 160 beats per minute. Most offices use an electronic Doppler device to check the baby's heartbeat. With this method, the baby's heartbeat sounds sort of like horses galloping inside the womb.

❀ **Starting sometime after 14 to 16 weeks, a nurse or doctor measures your fundal height.** In this procedure, a nurse or doctor uses a tape measure or her hands to measure your uterus, as shown in Figure 2-1. The idea is to get a rough idea about how the baby is growing and whether you have an adequate amount of amniotic fluid. Technically speaking, she is measuring the *fundal height* — the distance from the top of the pubic bone to the top of the uterus (called the *fundus*). By 20 weeks, the fundus usually reaches the level of the naval. After 20 weeks, the height in centimeters roughly equals the number of weeks pregnant you are.

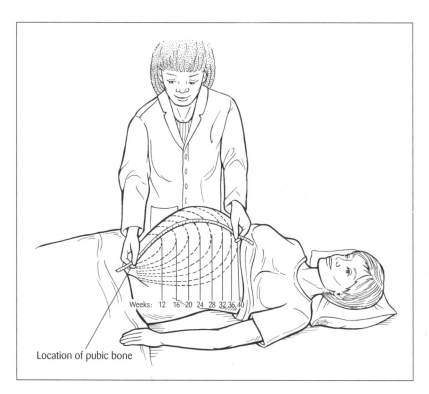

Weeks: 12 16 20 24 28 32 36 40

Location of pubic bone

Figure 2-1: Measuring fundal height to check that the baby is growing properly.

13

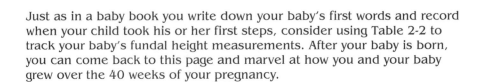

Just as in a baby book you write down your baby's first words and record when your child took his or her first steps, consider using Table 2-2 to track your baby's fundal height measurements. After your baby is born, you can come back to this page and marvel at how you and your baby grew over the 40 weeks of your pregnancy.

Table 2-2 Fundal Height Measurements

Date	Weeks into the Pregnancy	Measurement

A Look at the Effects of Medications, Alcohol, and Drugs on Your Baby

During your pregnancy, you'll probably experience at least a headache or two and an occasional case of heartburn. The question of whether you can safely take pain relievers, antacids, and other over-the-counter medicines is bound to come up. So, at your first prenatal visit, go over with your practitioner what medications are okay to take during pregnancy. Also be sure to talk about the effects of alcohol and smoking on your baby.

Taking medications

Exposure to the following drugs and chemicals is considered safe during pregnancy: acetaminophen, acyclovir, antiemetics (for example, phenothiazines and trimethobenzamide), antihistamines, aspartame (brand names Nutrasweet and Equal), low-dose aspirin, minor tranquilizers, penicillin, and zidovudine.

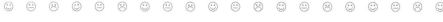

Here are a variety of medications that pregnant women often ask about:

❊ **Antiseizure drugs:** Some medicines for epileptic seizures are safer than others. Consult your doctor.

❊ **Birth control pills:** Yes, you can get pregnant when you're on the Pill. Oral contraceptives have shown no ill effects on babies in the womb.

❊ **Blood thinners:** One type of blood thinner, coumadine, can cause miscarriage, impair the baby's growth, or cause the baby to develop bleeding problems.

❊ **Drugs for high blood pressure:** A few of these medications can be problematic. Consult your doctor.

❊ **Ibuprofen (Advil, Motrin):** The occasional use of these and other NSAIDs (nonsteroidal anti-inflammatory drugs) is okay, but avoid using them habitually because they affect platelet function and the blood vessels in the baby's circulatory system.

❊ **Tetracycline:** If you take this antibiotic during the last several months of pregnancy, your baby's teeth may turn yellow.

❊ **Vitamin A:** This vitamin and some of its derivatives can cause miscarriage or birth defects. Discontinue using these drugs — the most common is the anti-acne drug Accutane — at least one month before trying to conceive.

Smoking

Unless you've been living on Mars for the past ten years, you no doubt are aware that smoking is a health risk. When you smoke, you run the risk of developing lung cancer, emphysema, and heart disease, among other illnesses. During pregnancy, however, smoking poses risks to your baby, as well. The carbon monoxide in cigarette smoke decreases the amount of oxygen that is delivered to a baby and cuts back on blood flow to the fetus. Smoking during pregnancy is associated with a greater risk of preterm delivery, miscarriage, placenta previa, placental abruption, preterm rupture of the amniotic membranes, and even sudden infant death syndrome after the baby is born.

Drinking alcohol

This topic is one that really needs to be put into perspective. Clearly, pregnant women who abuse alcohol put their babies at risk of *fetal alcohol syndrome,* which encompasses a wide variety of birth defects. The contro-versy arises because medical science hasn't been able to define an absolute safe level of alcohol intake during pregnancy. Scientific data shows that daily drinking or heavy binge drinking can lead to serious com-plications, but no studies indicate that an occasional glass of wine or an occasional drink causes harm to your baby. Moderation and common sense should be your guidelines. Some practitioners advise their patients to avoid alcohol during the first trimester, when the baby's organ systems are forming, and after that to limit their alcohol consumption to one to two drinks per week, but ask your practitioner and follow his or her advice.

Lifestyle Changes during Pregnancy

Your lifestyle will inevitably change during the nine months of your preg-nancy. You may wonder whether it's still okay to do some of the things you may have been used to doing on a regular basis before you were pregnant. This section provides information on these small changes.

❋ **Pampering yourself with beauty treatments:** Facials, manicures and pedicures from a reputable nail salon, leg and bikini waxes, and massages are all safe during pregnancy, and they may make you feel great! A few other beauty treatments, however, are cause for concern:

   Wrinkle creams: The two most common anti-wrinkle creams, Retin-A and Renova, both contain vitamin A derivatives, and data suggest that oral medications containing vitamin A derivatives (for example, Accutane) can cause birth defects. However, information that's avail-able on topical preparations such as over-the-counter Retin-A and Renova doesn't indicate any problems (prescription Retin-A is another story and should not be used). Due to the significant effects of oral preparations, however, many practitioners are reluctant to recommend any medications containing these compounds — oral or topical — to their patients.

   Chemical peels: Alpha-hydroxy acids are the main ingredients in chemical peels. The chemicals work topically, but small amounts are absorbed into the system. Scientists so far have been unable to find any data on whether chemical peels are safe during pregnancy. They're probably okay, but you may want to discuss this first with your practitioner.

   Hair dye: Practitioners tend to disagree about whether hair dyes are bad for babies, so you may want to stick to vegetable hair dyes. However, no evidence suggests that hair dyes today cause birth defects or miscarriage. Years ago, some of them contained formaldehyde and other potentially dangerous chemicals that could harm a baby, but the newer dyes don't contain these chemicals.

Hair perms: No scientific evidence suggests that the chemicals in hair permanents are harmful to a developing baby. These preparations usually do contain significant amounts of ammonia, however, and for your own safety, they should be used in well-ventilated areas.

❀ **Going into hot tubs, whirlpools, saunas, and steam rooms:** Using hot tubs, whirlpools, saunas, and steam rooms when you're pregnant can be risky on account of the high temperatures. Studies suggest that pregnant women whose core body temperatures rise significantly (above 102°) during the early weeks of pregnancy stand an increased risk of miscarriage or having babies with neural tube defects (spina bifida, for example). In general, soaking in a warm (not hot), soothing bath is fine, however.

❀ **Traveling:** The main potential problem with traveling during pregnancy is the distance it puts between you and your prenatal care provider. If you're close to your due date or if yours is a high-risk pregnancy, you probably shouldn't travel far from home. If your pregnancy is uncomplicated, travel during the first, second, and early third trimesters is usually okay. On long trips, get up and walk around every couple of hours. In a car, wear your seat belt below your abdomen, not above it, and keep the shoulder strap in its usual position. Most airlines allow women to fly if they're less than 36 weeks pregnant, but, just in case, carry a note from your practitioner indicating that he or she sees no medical reason why you shouldn't fly. Flying is perfectly safe, including using Dramamine in normal doses for airsickness and going through metal detectors.

❀ **Considering occupational hazards:** Should you continue working during pregnancy? Unfortunately, this question doesn't have a simple answer, because jobs are too diverse. Stress-free, sedentary jobs are perfectly safe (and no, computer terminals don't emit harmful electromagnetic fields). On the other hand, occupations that are physically demanding can be problematic, so you should talk to your practitioner.

❀ **Getting dental care:** You'll probably visit your dentist at least once during your pregnancy. If you need routine dental work — cavities filled, teeth pulled, crowns placed — don't worry. Local anesthesia and most pain medications are safe, but be sure to inform your dentist that you're pregnant. In addition, most antibiotics that dentists recommend for some dental work are also safe during pregnancy, but you should check with your practitioner to be sure. Even dental X-rays pose no significant problem for the fetus, as long as a lead apron is placed over your abdomen.

Half of all pregnant women develop a condition called *pregnancy gingivitis,* which is simply a reddening of the gums caused by this increased blood flow. In this condition, gums have a tendency to bleed easily, so be gentle when you brush and floss your teeth daily.

☺ ☺ ☹ ☺ ☺ ☹ ☺ ☺ ☹ ☺ ☺ ☹ ☺ ☺ ☹ ☺ ☺ ☺ ☹ ☺

❀ **Having sex:** For most couples, having sex during pregnancy is perfectly safe. In fact, some couples find that sex during pregnancy is better than before. In the first half of pregnancy, because your body hasn't changed noticeably, sex can usually continue as before. You may notice that your breasts are particularly sensitive to the touch, or even tender. Later, as the uterus grows, some sexual positions become more difficult. You and your partner may have to be a little creative in making things work. A lot of women ask us if it's still okay to have sex at the end of pregnancy, even if the cervix is a little bit dilated. It is perfectly fine as long as your membranes haven't ruptured (your water hasn't broken).

Most practitioners suggest refraining from intercourse if you are at a high risk for preterm labor because intercourse could introduce an infection into the uterus and because semen contains substances that are known to make the uterus contract.

Chapter 3

Diet and Exercise for the Expectant Mom

Throughout the ages, women have received all kinds of advice about what to eat while they're expecting. Cultural traditions, religious beliefs, and scientific thinking all have had their influence. As recently as a generation ago, women were told to limit how much they ate and drank to keep their weight gain to a minimum. At other times, they were encouraged to eat fatty foods, the idea being that the greater the weight gain, the healthier the child. These days, your practitioner's advice is likely to depend on your health habits and your weight when your pregnancy begins. This chapter provides you with the information you need to properly nourish yourself and your baby. It describes a proper diet and looks into exercise programs that are safe and healthy for pregnant women.

Choosing the Proper Diet

If your diet is balanced and not too heavy in sugar or fat, you don't need to modify the way you eat dramatically. During pregnancy, you should take in roughly 300 *extra* calories a day, on average. For example, if you're at a healthy weight and you're taking in 2,100 calories per day, while pregnant you should take in an average of 2,400 calories per day (perhaps a little less during your first trimester and a little more during your third).

Where are you going to get the extra 300 calories a day you need during pregnancy? You could stop off for a double cheeseburger and fries (actually, that would put you well over 300). Or you could opt for low-fat yogurt or cottage cheese. You can see which choice is wiser. The key is to make sure that your extra calories are packed with nutrients, protein, and carbohydrates.

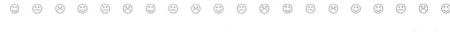
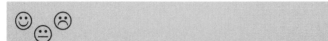

Is caffeine safe during pregnancy?

Some women think that caffeine is found only in coffee, but caffeine is found as well in many foods and beverages you eat and drink daily: tea, many sodas, cocoa, and chocolate. No evidence shows that caffeine causes birth defects, but if you consume caffeine in large amounts, you can raise the risk of low birth weight and miscarriage.

Most studies suggest that it takes more than 300 milligrams of caffeine a day to affect the fetus. The average cup of coffee – the *average* cup, no the super-mondo – has between 100 and 150 milligrams of caffeine. So drinking up to two average-sized cups of coffee per day is usually okay during pregnancy.

 No single food can satisfy all of your important nutritional needs. The food pyramid from the USDA, shown in Figure 3-1, is a general guideline that illustrates how much food from each group you should eat. Eat less from the food groups at the top of the pyramid and more from the food groups at the bottom.

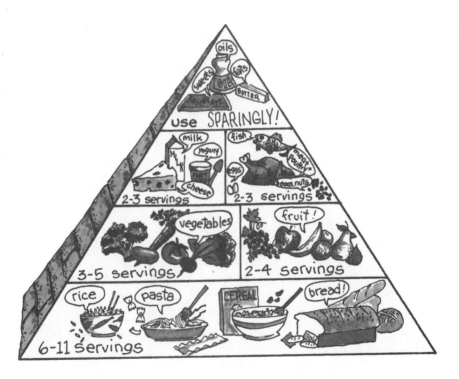

Figure 3-1: Use the food pyramid to help you eat healthy during pregnancy.

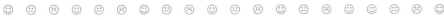
Here are the other dietary concerns to consider when you are pregnant:

❀ **Water:** As your pregnancy progresses, your body needs a lot of extra fluid. Early on, some women who don't drink enough liquid feel weak or faint. Later in pregnancy, dehydration can lead to premature contractions. Make a point of drinking plenty of water — about six to eight glasses a day.

❀ **Vitamins:** If your diet is healthy and balanced, you get most of the vitamins and minerals you need naturally — with the exception of iron, folic acid, and calcium. To make sure that you get enough of these nutrients and as insurance against inadequate eating habits, your practitioner is likely to recommend prenatal vitamins.

❀ **Folic acid:** In the past decade, folic acid has become a nutritional requirement for all pregnant women. *Folate,* as it is also known, reduces the occurrence of birth defects of the brain and spinal cord. Today, all women considering pregnancy are advised to consume 0.4 milligrams of folic acid every day, starting 30 days before conception.

❀ **Iron:** You need more iron when you're expecting, because both you and the baby are making new red blood cells every day. On average, you need 30 milligrams of extra iron every day of your pregnancy, which is what most prenatal vitamins contain. Blood counts can easily drop during pregnancy, as your body gradually makes more and more blood *plasma* (fluid) and *relatively* fewer red blood cells (what is called a *dilutional anemia*). Foods rich in iron include chicken, fish, red meat, green leafy vegetables, and enriched or whole-grain breads and cereals.

❀ **Calcium:** You need about 1,200 milligrams of calcium every day while you're pregnant. If you are already starting out somewhat calcium deficient, the calcium requirements of the developing baby will only make matters worse for you. A fetus is able to extract enough calcium from its mother, even if it means getting it at the expense of the mother's bones. So the extra calcium needed during pregnancy is really aimed at protecting you and your health. Getting enough calcium from your diet alone is possible if you really pay attention. You can get it from three to four servings of calcium-rich foods — such as milk, yogurt, cheese, green leafy vegetables, and canned fish with bones (if your stomach can take it). Supermarkets also stock special lactose-free foods that are high in calcium.

 If your diet is low in calcium, take a supplement. Tums and some other antacids contain quite a bit of calcium and, at the same time, they help relieve any pregnancy heartburn you may have. (A single Tums tablet has the equivalent calcium content of an 8-ounce glass of milk.)

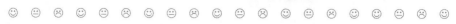
 Women commonly experience morning sickness during the first trimester (the first three months, which are discussed in Chapter 4). If you're experiencing this nausea and are unable to eat a well-balanced diet, you may wonder whether or not you are getting enough nutrition for you and the baby. The fact is, you can go for several weeks not eating an optimal diet without any ill effects on the baby. You may find that the only foods you can tolerate are foods heavy in starch or carbohydrates. If all you feel like eating are potatoes, bread, and pasta, go right ahead. It is more important that you keep something down rather than starve.

Getting Enough Exercise

The great fitness movement has not left pregnant women behind. You see women in all stages of pregnancy jogging in parks, working out in gyms, or stretching limbs in yoga classes.

Where does the weight go?

The good news is, the weight you gain during pregnancy doesn't all go to your thighs. Then again, it doesn't all go to the baby. A pregnant woman typically adds a little to her own body fat. It's a myth, however, that you can tell by a woman's pattern of weight gain – more in the hips or more in the belly – whether she's going to have a boy or a girl. The following list gives you a realistic view of what you're gaining – assuming a total weight gain of 27 pounds, which is fairly average.

* Amniotic fluid: 2 pounds
* Body water: 4 pounds
* Breasts: 1 pound
* Extra blood: 3 pounds
* Fat stores: 7 pounds
* Fetus: 7 pounds
* Placenta: 1 pound
* Uterus: 2 pounds

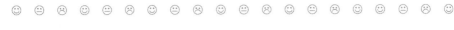

During pregnancy, exercise helps your body in two ways: It keeps your heart strong and your muscles in shape, and it relieves the basic discomforts of pregnancy. Studies show that the earlier in pregnancy a woman gets regular exercise, the more comfortable she is likely to feel throughout the nine months. Some evidence shows that regular exercise makes for shorter labor, too. It can even help alleviate the symptoms of diabetes. So if you're in good health and not at risk for obstetrical or medical complications, by all means go ahead and continue with your exercise program — unless your program calls for climbing Mount Fuji, entering a professional boxing match, or some other super-strenuous activity. It's a good idea to go over your exercise program with your practitioner, so he or she knows what you are doing, and so that you can ask any questions you have.

Adapting to changes in your body

Even if you work out in moderation, keep in mind that pregnancy causes your body to undergo real physical changes, which can affect your strength, stamina, and performance. The following list details some of those changes:

❋ **Cardiovascular changes:** When you're pregnant, the amount of blood that your heart pumps through your body increases. That increase in blood volume usually has no effect on your workout. But if you lie flat on your back, especially after about 16 weeks of pregnancy, you may feel dizzy, faint, or even nauseous. Known as the *supine hypotension syndrome*, this dizziness sometimes happens when the enlarging uterus presses down on major blood vessels that return blood to the heart, thus decreasing the heart's output. It happens even more readily if you're carrying twins (or more), because your uterus is that much heavier.

If you're doing any exercises that require you to lie on your back (and also if you're accustomed to sleeping on your back), put a small pillow or foam wedge under the right side of your back or your right hip. This tilts you slightly sidewise and effectively lifts your uterus off the blood vessels.

❋ **Respiratory changes:** Your body is using more oxygen than usual to support the growing baby. At the same time, breathing is more work than it used to be because your enlarging uterus presses upward against your diaphragm. For some women, this difficulty makes performing aerobic exercise a little harder.

☺ ☻ ☹ ☺ ☻ ☹ ☺ ☻ ☹ ☺ ☻ ☹ ☺ ☻ ☹ ☺ ☻ ☹ ☺

❀ **Structural changes:** As your body shape changes — bigger abdomen, larger breasts — your center of gravity shifts, which can affect your balance. You notice it especially if you dance, bicycle, ski, surf, ride horses, or do anything else (walk tightropes, maybe?) where balance is important. In addition, hormones cause some laxness in your joints, which also can make balance more difficult and may increase your risk of injury.

❀ **Metabolic changes:** Pregnant women use up carbohydrates faster than non-pregnant women do, which means that they are at a higher risk of developing *hypoglycemia* (or low blood sugar). Exercise can be very useful in helping lower and control blood sugar levels, but it also increases the body's need for carbohydrates. So if you exercise, make extra sure that you're eating an adequate amount of carbs.

❀ **Effects on the uterus:** One study of women at *term* (far enough along to deliver) showed that their contractions increased after moderate aerobic exercise. Another study indicated that exercise is associated with a lower risk of early labor. But most studies have shown that exercise has no effect either way and that exercise does not pose a risk of preterm labor in healthy pregnant women.

❀ **Effect on birth weight:** Some studies have shown that women who work out strenuously during pregnancy have lighter-weight babies. The same effect appears to occur in women who perform heavy physical work in a standing position while they're pregnant. But this decrease in birth weight seems to be due mainly to a decrease in the newborn's subcutaneous fat. In other words, more exercise has no effect on the fetus's normal growth.

Workout guide

No matter what your particular exercise regimen is, keep in mind the basic rules for working out during pregnancy. The following is a list of tips to consider when keeping up activities as your baby grows larger and larger:

❀ If you have a moderate exercise routine, keep it up. If you've been pretty sedentary, don't suddenly plunge into a strenuous program; ease in slowly. Keeping up a regular schedule of moderate activity is better than engaging in infrequent spurts of intense exercise.

❀ Avoid overheating, especially during the first six weeks of pregnancy.

❀ Avoid exercising flat on your back for long periods of time; doing so may reduce blood flow to your heart.

☺ ☺ ☹ ☺ ☺ ☺ ☹ ☺ ☺ ☹ ☺ ☺ ☹ ☺ ☺ ☹ ☺ ☺ ☺ ☹ ☺

❀ Try not to beat yourself up if you find that pregnancy makes it harder to continue the workout routine you're accustomed to. Modify your program according to what you can reasonably tolerate. Listen to your body. If weight-lifting suddenly hurts your back, lighten up. You may have an easier time performing non-weight-bearing exercises like swimming or bicycling.

❀ Watch how your center of gravity shifts. You probably should avoid surfing, horseback riding, skiing, or any other sport that can cause injury if you're out of balance. Also avoid anything that puts you at risk of being hurt in the abdomen, as well as high-impact, bouncy exercises that can tax your loosening joints.

❀ Carry a bottle of water to every exercise session and stay well hydrated.

❀ Eat a well-balanced diet that includes an adequate supply of carbohydrates.

❀ Talk to your practitioner about what your peak exercise heart rate should be. (Many practitioners suggest 140 beats per minute as the upper limit, but this isn't a hard and fast rule anymore.) Then regularly measure your heart rate at the peak of your workout to make sure that it's at a safe level.

Reasons not to exercise

As good as exercise is for most pregnant women, it's not advisable for everyone. If you have any of the following conditions, you may be better off not working out – at least not until you discuss the situation with your doctor:

❀ Bleeding

❀ Incompetent cervix

❀ Intrauterine growth restriction

❀ Low volume of amniotic fluid

❀ Placenta previa (late in pregnancy)

❀ Pregnancy-induced hypertension

❀ Premature labor or preterm rupture of the membranes

❀ Triplets or more

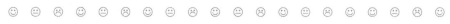

 By using Table 3-1, you can keep track of how often you exercise during your pregnancy. Starting at Week 1 and continuing through Week 40, write in the number of minutes you exercise for each day. This table allows you and your practitioner to see how often you exercise and whether you are getting enough.

Table 3-1 Exercise Chart

Week	Mon	Tues	Wed	Thurs	Fri	Sat	Sun
1							
2							
3							
4							
5							
6							
7							
8							
9							
10							
11							
12							
13							
14							
15							
16							
17							
18							
19							
20							

☺ ☻ ☹ ☺ ☻ ☹ ☺ ☻ ☹ ☺ ☻ ☹ ☺ ☻ ☹ ☺ ☺ ☻ ☹ ☺

Week	Mon	Tues	Wed	Thurs	Fri	Sat	Sun
21							
22							
23							
24							
25							
26							
27							
28							
29							
30							
31							
32							
33							
34							
35							
36							
37							
38							
39							
40							

Stop exercising — and talk to your doctor — if you experience any of the following symptoms:

❀ Shortness of breath out of proportion to the exercise you are doing

❀ Vaginal bleeding

❀ Rapid heartbeat (that is, more than 140 beats per minute)

❀ Dizziness or feeling faint

❀ Any significant pain

☺ ☺ ☹ ☺ ☺ ☹ ☺ ☺ ☹ ☺ ☺ ☹ ☺ ☺ ☹ ☺ ☺ ☺ ☹ ☺

Part 2

What's Happening to Me?

As you become more calendar-conscious, you find out that pregnancy lasts roughly 40 weeks, or a little longer than 9 months. Because that can seem like an awfully long time, perhaps the most useful way to think of pregnancy is to divide it, as doctors have always done, into three trimesters.

The baby's growth and the changes that occur in your body happen in three fairly distinct stages, each one lasting three months, or one trimester. Not coincidentally, this part is similarly divided into three chapters. Chapter 4 covers the first trimester; Chapter 5, the second; and Chapter 6, the third.

Chapter 4

Put One Foot in Front of the Other: The First Trimester

In This Chapter

☺ Understanding how your baby develops in the womb

☺ Being prepared for the physical changes that pregnancy brings

☺ Anticipating tests and questions at your prenatal visits

☺ Understanding diagnostic tests and when they are necessary

☺ Recognizing when problems occur

The first trimester of your pregnancy is an exhilarating time, but it's also a time for nervousness and apprehension, especially if you've never been pregnant before.

You've embarked on a wonderful journey, and this chapter covers what to expect in the first three months of your journey. This chapter helps you understand the development of your fetus and the changes that you see in your body. You find out what happens at your first prenatal visit and the visits that follow in your first trimester. You also get information on diagnostic tests that may be performed during your first trimester and let you know why these tests are necessary and whether they pose any risks. Finally, you discover when you have reason to be concerned and call your practitioner — and when to take a deep breath and relax.

A New Life Takes Shape

Over the next three months, exciting changes happen inside your body and to your body. To help you understand them, this section offers a short biology lesson. Don't worry, you won't be quizzed on this material, but understanding the female reproductive system helps you understand how your baby develops inside your body and what you will undergo during the next several months.

Part 2: What's Happening to Me?

☺ ☺ ☹ ☺ ☹ ☹ ☺ ☹ ☹ ☺ ☹ ☹ ☺ ☺ ☹ ☹ ☺ ☺ ☹ ☹ ☺

Figure 4-1 shows the biology of the female reproductive system. Pregnancy begins when the egg and sperm meet in the fallopian tube and form a *zygote* — a single cell. Very shortly, this single cell starts dividing and turns into a *blastocyst.* The blastocyst travels down the fallopian tube to the *uterus,* better known as the womb. At this point you and your baby begin to experience major changes. At about the fifth day of development, in what is known as *implantation,* the blastocyst attaches to the blood-rich lining of the uterus. Part of the blastocyst becomes the *embryo,* the term for a baby in the first eight weeks of development, and the other part becomes the *placenta.*

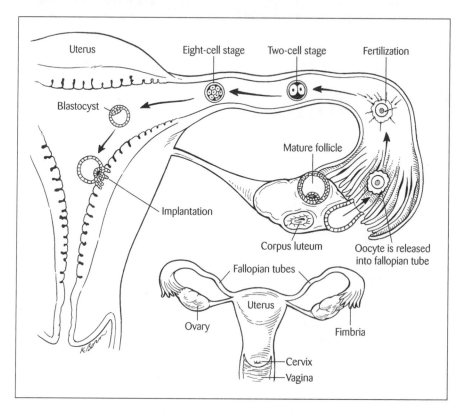

Figure 4-1: The female reproductive system in action.

Soon after the embryo implants in the uterus, the placenta begins to form. Although they don't mix, the mother's blood and baby's blood come into close contact inside the placenta. This allows the mother and baby to transfer different substances — nutrients, oxygen, and waste — back and forth. Like a tree, the placenta forms large branches called *villi,* and these branches, in turn, divide into smaller and smaller branches. Eventually,

☺ ☻ ☹ ☺ ☻ ☹ ☺ ☻ ☹ ☺ ☻ ☹ ☺ ☻ ☹ ☺ ☺ ☻ ☹ ☺

small fetal blood vessels form on the tiniest branches of the placenta, and, about three weeks after fertilization, these blood vessels join to form the baby's circulatory system. Now the baby's heart begins to beat.

Your baby grows within the *amniotic sac* in the uterus. To understand what an amniotic sac is, imagine a baby developing inside a balloon, only instead of the balloon being filled with air, it's filled with clear fluid called the *amniotic fluid.* The balloon itself is composed of two thin layers of membrane, the *chorion* and *amnion.* These membranes line the inner walls of the uterus. When doctors and midwives talk about "breaking the bag of water," they are referring to what happens when these membranes are ruptured. In the uterus, the baby "swims" in the amniotic fluid and is attached to the placenta by the umbilical cord.

Figure 4-2 shows a diagram of an early pregnancy, including a developing fetus and the *cervix.* The cervix is the opening to the uterus. It opens up, or *dilates,* when you are in labor (see Chapter 7).

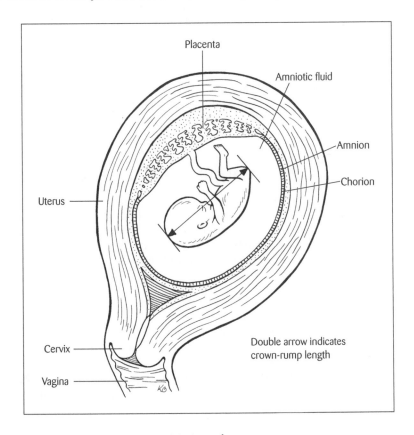

Figure 4-2: An early pregnancy.

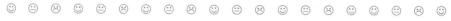
In the eighth week of pregnancy, the developing embryo becomes a *fetus*. Amazingly, almost all of the baby's major organs and structures are already formed by this time. In the remaining 32 weeks, the fetus's structures will grow and mature.

By the end of the second month, arms, legs, fingers, and toes begin to form, and the fetus begins to perform small, spontaneous movements. During an ultrasound examination (discussed in the "Ultrasound" section later in this chapter) in the first trimester, you can see these movements on the screen. The brain grows rapidly. Ears and eyes appear. The external genitalia emerge, although sex differences still can't be detected by ultrasound.

By the end of the third month, the fetus is about 4 inches long and weighs about 1 ounce. The head looks large and round. The intestines, which protrude slightly into the umbilical cord during week 10, are now well inside the abdomen. Fingernails appear. Hair begins to grow on the baby's head. The kidneys start working. Between 9 and 12 weeks, the fetus begins to produce urine, which can be seen within the small fetal bladder on ultrasound.

 The word "weeks" throughout this book means menstrual weeks, or how many weeks have passed since the last menstrual period, not how many weeks have passed since conception. So at eight weeks, a baby is really six weeks from conception.

How Your Body Changes during Pregnancy

Not that you need reminding, but your baby isn't the only one growing and changing during pregnancy. Your body also has to adjust, and the adjustments it makes are not necessarily pleasant or comfortable. On the idea that being prepared for what lies ahead can help ease your mind, this section explains what's in store for you during the first trimester.

Breast changes

One of the earliest and most amazing changes in your body happens to your breasts. As early as the first month of pregnancy, most women notice their breasts growing considerably larger and feeling very tender. The nipples and *areolae* (the circular areas around the nipples) grow bigger and

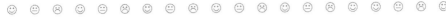

may begin to darken. These changes are caused by the large amounts of estrogen and progesterone that your body produces during pregnancy. The glands inside your breasts are growing and branching out in preparation for milk production and breast-feeding. You may also notice large, bluish blood vessels as the blood supply to your breasts increases markedly.

Plan to go through several bra sizes while you're pregnant — and don't skimp on new bras. Good breast support helps reduce stretching and sagging later on.

Fatigue

During the first trimester, you will likely feel overwhelming fatigue, a side effect of the physical changes your body is experiencing, including the dramatic rise in hormone levels. Take comfort from knowing that the exhaustion you feel will probably go away in the 12th to 14th week of pregnancy. As your fatigue lessens, you'll feel more energetic and almost normal, until about 30 to 34 weeks into your pregnancy, when you may start getting tired again. Fatigue is nature's way of telling you to get more rest. Try to catch a short nap during the day and go to bed earlier than usual at night.

Any-time-of-day sickness

For some women, the nausea that can strike during the first trimester is worse in the morning, maybe because the stomach is empty then. But ask anyone who's had morning sickness, and she'll tell you that it can hit at any time. Any-time-of-day sickness often starts during the fifth or sixth week of pregnancy — that is, three to four weeks after you miss your period — and goes away, or at least becomes milder, by the end of the 11th or 12th week. It can last longer, though, particularly in women who are expecting twins, because multiple placentas release more hCG (human chorionic gonadotropin), the hormone that is believed to cause morning sickness.

Even when nausea doesn't actually cause you to vomit, it can be extremely uncomfortable and truly debilitating. Certain odors — from foods, perfumes, or musty places — can make it worse. If your queasiness gets out of control, you experience weight loss, you can't keep food or liquids down, or you feel dizzy or faint, call your doctor.

Keeping nausea at bay

Although these tips don't make nausea disappear completely, they can help keep it at bay:

* Eat small, frequent meals, so that your stomach is never empty.

* Don't worry too much about sticking to a balanced diet; just eat whatever appeals to you during this relatively short period of time. You might try eating dry toast, whole wheat crackers, potatoes, and other bland, easy-to-digest carbohydrates.

* Keep crackers by your bedside. Some women find that eating them before getting out of bed in the morning helps against nausea.

* If taking your prenatal vitamins makes the symptoms worse, try taking them at night just before you go to bed. If they still cause nausea, skip them for a few days. If you're less than six weeks pregnant, you can take folic acid instead of your prenatal vitamin. Folic acid is the main supplement that you need early in your pregnancy, and it's much less likely to upset your stomach than a multivitamin.

* Try vitamin B_6. Evidence suggests that 25 milligrams of this nutrient three times a day can reduce queasiness. But talk to your doctor before starting a B_6 regimen.

* Ginger helps some women. Take it in the form of tea or tablets.

* If nausea worsens when you brush your teeth, try switching toothpaste brands.

* If you are bothered by the accumulation of saliva in your mouth, sucking on lemon drop candies may help.

* Try acupressure wrist bands, which are sold in drugstores and health food stores and give some women relief. Relaxation exercises and even hypnosis also work for some women.

* Avoid perfume counters, kitchens where spicy or fried foods are being prepared, smelly taxi cabs, barnyards, or other places where odors are strong.

* For extreme nausea, talk to your doctor about prescription medicines or other over-the-counter medicines.

Bloating

Well before the baby is big enough to stretch out your stomach, your belt may feel tighter, and your belly may look bloated and distended. *Progesterone*, one of two key pregnancy hormones, makes you retain water and slows down your bowels, causing them to enlarge and increase the size of your abdomen. *Estrogen*, the other key hormone, causes your uterus to enlarge, which also makes your abdomen feel bigger.

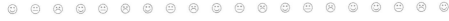

Frequent urination

Starting early in pregnancy, some women feel as if they're spending all their time in the restroom. Toward the end of your first trimester, your uterus expands and rises into the abdominal cavity. This shift may compress your bladder, which both decreases its capacity and increases the feeling that you need to urinate. Because blood volume rises markedly during pregnancy, the rate at which your kidneys produce urine also increases. And because drinking plenty of fluids during pregnancy is necessary to avoid dehydration, you urinate more, anyway.

Headaches

Many pregnant women get headaches more often than they used to. Nausea, fatigue, hunger, the normal physiologic decrease in blood pressure that starts to occur at this time, tension, and even depression can cause a headache. Food and extra rest can usually cure headaches that are caused by nausea, fatigue, or hunger, but if neither of these tactics works or your headaches are chronic or recurrent, you may need to take medications, despite their effect on your fetus. Taking acetaminophen (such as Tylenol) or ibuprofen (such as Motrin) in recommended doses is perfectly okay for headache relief, but avoid taking regular doses of aspirin, because adult doses of aspirin can affect platelet function (important in blood clotting). If over-the-counter medications don't relieve your headache, talk to a health practitioner about taking a mild tranquilizer or anti-migraine medication.

Be sure to consult your practitioner before taking any medication. Later in pregnancy, severe and unremitting headaches may signal the onset of a condition called preeclampsia. In that case, your headache may be accompanied by swelling in your hands and feet, as well as high blood pressure. If you suffer a severe headache in the late second or third trimester, call your practitioner. See Chapter 6 for details.

Constipation

Half of pregnant women complain of constipation. Large amounts of progesterone circulating in your bloodstream slow the activity of your digestive tract, and the iron in prenatal vitamins can make matters worse. Here are suggestions for dealing with constipation:

* **Eat plenty of high-fiber foods.** Bran cereals, fruits, and vegetables all are good sources of fiber. Some women find it helpful to eat popcorn, but choose the low-fat kind, without butter and added oil. Check the fiber content on package labels and choose foods with a high-fiber content.

37

☺ ☹ ☺ ☺ ☺ ☹ ☺ ☺ ☹ ☺ ☺ ☹ ☺ ☺ ☹ ☺ ☺ ☺ ☹ ☺

❊ **Drink plenty of water.** Staying well hydrated keeps food and waste moving through the digestive tract. Some juices, especially prune juice, may help, but others, such as apple juice can exacerbate the problem.

❊ **Take stool softeners.** A stool softener such as Colace (docusate sodium) is not a laxative — it just keeps the stool soft. Stool softeners are safe during pregnancy and may be taken two to three times a day. (Avoid laxatives, however, because they can cause abdominal cramping and, occasionally, uterine contractions.)

❊ **Exercise regularly.** Exercise is known to help constipation, so enjoy safe exercise, even if it's only walking. See Chapter 3 for more information.

If you are extremely constipated and not at risk for preterm labor, you may talk to your practitioner about the short-term use of a mild laxative such as a glycerin suppository.

Cramps

You may feel a vague, menstrual-like cramping sensation during the first trimester. Mild cramping is a common symptom and is nothing to be concerned about. The cramping is probably related to the uterus growing and enlarging. However, if you experience cramping along with vaginal bleeding, give your practitioner a call. Although the majority of women who experience bleeding and cramping go on to have perfectly normal pregnancies, these two symptoms appearing together are sometimes associated with miscarriage.

All about Prenatal Visits

Visits to your health practitioner should be a regular part of your pregnancy, not just to make sure *you* are healthy, but to make sure your baby is, too. Prenatal visits differ from annual checkups. In case you wonder what prenatal visits are like, what kind of examinations you will undergo, and what questions the health practitioner will ask, this section tells you everything you need to know to be prepared for prenatal visits during the first trimester.

Your first prenatal visit

After you discover you are pregnant, set up an appointment with a health practitioner. Your first prenatal visit usually lasts 40 minutes or more because the doctor has so much information to provide and so many topics to discuss. This initial visit may be your first with the practitioner

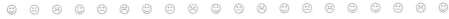
who will guide you through pregnancy. Or perhaps you have a long-standing relationship with an ob/gyn or family-practice doctor with whom you've already discussed topics that are typically covered at the initial prenatal visit. Whatever your situation, you're moving into new territory.

Consultation

During your first visit, your practitioner discusses with you your medical and obstetrical history. He or she asks about aspects of your physical health, as well as elements of your lifestyle that may affect your pregnancy:

- **Lifestyle:** You're asked general questions about your lifestyle. For example, you are asked whether you smoke, drink alcohol in immoderate amounts, have dietary restrictions, and exercise. Your practitioner asks about your occupation to find out whether your job requires you to be sedentary or active. Your practitioner asks whether you work nights or long shifts.

- **Date of your last menstrual period:** You are asked the start date of your last menstrual period to determine your due date. If you don't know precisely when your last period began, try to remember the date of conception. If you know neither of these dates, your practitioner may schedule an ultrasound exam to see how far along you are. (See the "Ultrasound" section later in this chapter for details on this procedure.)

- **Obstetrical and gynecological history:** You're asked about your obstetrical and gynecological history, whether you have been pregnant before, and whether you have any experiences with fibroid tumors, vaginal infections, and other gynecological problems. Your past history can help determine how best to manage this pregnancy.

- **Medical problems:** Your practitioner asks about any medical problems you have had, surgeries you have undergone, and allergies to medications.

- **Family medical histories:** You're asked about your family's medical history as well as the medical history of the baby's father. Your practitioner asks these questions to identify pregnancy-related conditions that can recur from generation to generation.

- **Ethnic roots:** Your practitioner asks about your and your partner's family histories to see whether your families are free of genetic disorders. Some genetic disorders occur more frequently in one ethnicity than others.

Physical exam

At your first prenatal visit, your practitioner examines your head, neck, breasts, heart, lungs, abdomen, and extremities. He or she also performs an internal pelvic exam, which evaluates your uterus, cervix, and ovaries, and he or she performs a Pap test.

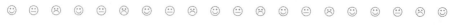
After the exam is a good time for you to discuss the overall plan for your pregnancy and talk about any possible problems. You can also discuss what medications you can take while you're pregnant, when you should call for help, and what tests you can expect to undergo throughout your pregnancy.

Blood tests

During your first prenatal visit, your practitioner needs to draw your blood for certain tests. The following tests are routine:

- **A standard test for blood type, Rh factor, and antibody status:** Determines whether your blood is type A, B, or O, and whether you are Rh-positive or Rh-negative. The antibody test is designed to tell whether special blood-group antibodies to certain antigens (such as the Rh antigen) are present in your blood.

- **Complete blood count (CBC):** Checks for *anemia,* which refers to a low blood count, as well as your *platelet count.* Platelets are a component of blood important in clotting.

- **VDRL:** Checks for *syphilis,* a venereal disease.

- **Hepatitis:** Checks for evidence of the hepatitis viruses. These viruses come in several different types. Hepatitis B can be present without producing any symptoms.

- **Rubella:** Checks for immunity to *rubella,* also called *German measles.* Most women have been vaccinated against rubella or carry antibodies against the disease because they had the illness in the past. If you are not immune to rubella, your health practitioner will counsel you to be very careful to avoid contact with anyone who has the illness. You will also be advised to get vaccinated against rubella soon after you deliver.

- **HIV:** Checks for the presence of HIV, the virus that causes AIDS. Most states require health care providers to ask whether you want to be checked for HIV. Medication is now available to reduce the risk of transmission to the baby, as well as slow disease progression in the mother. The HIV test can usually be performed at the same time as the other prenatal blood tests.

Doctors sometimes need to perform other tests, as well. You may undergo these additional tests:

- **Glucose screen:** Checks whether you are at a high risk of develop-ing *gestational diabetes.* This test is usually performed 24 to 28 weeks into pregnancy, but sometimes it is done in the first trimester. See Chapter 5 for more on diabetes.

- **Varicella:** Checks for immunity to *varicella,* also known as chicken pox. If you are not sure whether you had chicken pox or you are certain that you did not have it, tell your practitioner. This way, you can be tested for immunity.

🌸 **Toxoplasmosis:** Checks for immunity to *toxoplasmosis,* a type of parasitic infection. In the United States, testing for toxoplasmosis is not done routinely unless you are at a high risk for toxoplasmosis. If you have an outdoor cat and you are the one who changes the litter box, your practitioner is likely to test for toxoplasmosis.

🌸 **Cytomegalovirus (CMV):** Tests for a CMV infection, a common childhood infection. If you often come in contact with school-age children who may have the infection, your practitioner may suggest taking this test.

Urine tests

Each time you visit your practitioner during your pregnancy, including the first prenatal visit, you are asked to leave a sample of urine. The urine sample is needed in order to check for the presence of glucose (for a possible sign of diabetes), and protein (for evidence of preeclampsia).

Ultrasound

Your practitioner may suggest undergoing a first-trimester ultrasound exam. In an ultrasound exam, sound waves create a picture of the uterus and the baby inside it. If the exam is performed *transvaginally,* a probe called a *transducer* is inserted in the vagina. This technique offers the advantage of examining the uterus more closely and getting a better picture of the fetus than a *transabdominal* (through the abdomen) ultrasound examination. Ultrasound examinations do not involve radiation. Some women worry that inserting a probe in the vagina will harm the baby, but the procedure is perfectly safe.

The following are evaluated during a first-trimester ultrasound exam:

🌸 **The accuracy of your due date:** Your practitioner can tell whether the fetus is larger or smaller than the date suggested by your last menstrual period. If the *crown-rump length* — the length of the fetus from the crown of the head to the rump — is more than three or four days removed from your due date, your doctor may change your due date. An ultrasound in the first trimester is a more accurate means of confirming or establishing the due date than an ultrasound performed later on.

🌸 **Fetal viability:** An ultrasound examination performed five to six weeks after conception should be able to detect a fetal heartbeat. After a fetal heartbeat has been identified, the risk of miscarriage drops significantly, to about 3 percent. Prior to five weeks, the fetus itself may not be visible; instead, the ultrasound may show only the gestational sac.

⊙ ☺ ⊗ ⊙ ⊖ ⊗ ⊙ ⊖ ⊗ ⊙ ⊖ ⊗ ⊙ ⊖ ⊗ ⊙ ⊙ ⊖ ⊗ ⊙

* **Fetal abnormalities:** Although a complete ultrasound examination to detect structural abnormalities in the fetus is usually not performed until 20 weeks, some problems may already be visible by 11 to 12 weeks. Much of the brain, spine, limbs, abdomen, and urinary tract structures may be seen in a transvaginal ultrasound examination.

* **Fetal number:** An ultrasound shows whether you are carrying more than one fetus.

* **The condition of your ovaries:** An ultrasound can reveal cysts or other abnormalities in your ovaries. Whether removal of these cysts is necessary depends on the size of the cyst and any symptoms you may be having.

* **The presence of fibroid tumors:** Also called *fibroids*, these are benign overgrowths of the muscle of the uterus.

* **Location of the pregnancy:** Occasionally, the pregnancy is located outside the uterus. This is called an *ectopic pregnancy* (see the "Ectopic pregnancy" section later in this chapter).

Routine prenatal visits

Your first prenatal visit is usually 40 minutes or so, but subsequent visits are usually much shorter, sometimes only 5 to 10 minutes long. How often you visit your practitioner depends on your particular needs and whether special risk factors pertain to you. In general, prenatal visits are scheduled every four weeks during the first trimester. At these visits, the practitioner checks your urine, your blood pressure, your weight, and the baby's heartbeat.

Causes for Concern in the First Trimester

In each trimester, a few things may go less than smoothly. In the first trimester, bleeding, miscarriage, ectopic pregnancy, and ovarian torsion are the primary concerns. The following sections describe these conditions and what they may mean to you.

Bleeding

Early in the first trimester, about the time of your missed period, a little bleeding from the vagina is not uncommon. This is called *implantation bleeding.* About one-third of women experience bleeding during the first trimester; it occurs when the fertilized egg attaches to the lining of the uterus. The amount of blood is usually less than the amount from a period. Bleeding can last for one or two days. Sometimes women are confused by it and mistake implantation bleeding for a period. In general,

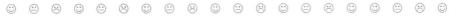
bright red bleeding indicates active bleeding, whereas dark staining indicates old blood that is making its way out from the cervix and vagina.

Miscarriage

About one in five pregnancies end in early miscarriage. In a miscarriage, bleeding is often accompanied by abdominal cramping — call your doctor as soon as you can. Unfortunately, most miscarriages can't be prevented. Many, if not most, are simply nature's way of handling an abnormal pregnancy. Miscarriage may lead to cramping and bleeding. You may feel abdominal pains that are stronger than menstrual cramps, and you may pass fetal and placental tissue. If you experience heavy bleeding and abnormally painful cramps, call your doctor. Bleeding, however, isn't necessarily a sign of miscarriage. As the preceding section explains, some bleeding is not uncommon.

Ectopic pregnancy

An *ectopic pregnancy* occurs when the fertilized egg implants outside the uterus — in one of the fallopian tubes, the ovary, the abdomen, or the cervix. An ectopic pregnancy is a serious threat to the mother's health. Fortunately, ultrasound has advanced to the point where it can detect ectopic pregnancies very early. Signs of an ectopic pregnancy include vaginal bleeding, abdominal pain, dizziness, and feeling faint. How your doctor treats the problem depends on the location of the embryo or fetus, how far along the pregnancy is, and the particular symptoms you are experiencing. Unfortunately, the embryo or fetus can't be moved to the uterus so that the pregnancy can continue as normal.

Ovarian torsion

An ovarian cyst may cause the ovary to twist and turn and cause what is called *ovarian torsion.* Ovarian torsion sometimes occurs in women who have taken fertility drugs. These women tend to have large ovaries and lots of follicles. The main symptom of ovarian torsion is excruciating pain, which may come and go on one side of the abdomen. If you experience these symptoms, call your doctor.

Part 2: What's Happening to Me?

Chapter 5

I've Never Felt So Good! The Second Trimester

The second trimester, which encompasses the three months between week 13 and week 26, is usually the most enjoyable part of pregnancy. The nausea and fatigue so common during the first trimester usually disappear. You feel more energetic. You start to understand what being pregnant is all about, and you're comfortable with it. Best of all, you feel the baby moving inside you. This is often the time you begin sharing your exciting news with family, friends, and co-workers.

This chapter spells out what your second trimester feels like. You find out more about changes you've begun to notice — from your baby's movements to changes in your skin and hair. You get the lowdown on ultrasounds, amniocentesis, and all the other medical tests you're given. Finally, this chapter alerts you to signs of possible trouble.

A Look at How the Baby Develops

As you can see in Figure 5-1, your baby grows rapidly during the second trimester, weeks 13 through 26. At 13 weeks, the fetus is about 3 inches (8 cm) long, but by 26 weeks, it's roughly 14 inches (35 cm) long and weighs about 2¼ pounds (1,022 grams). Between weeks 14 and 16, the limbs begin to look like arms and legs; in fact, coordinated arm and leg movements are observable on ultrasound (see the "Ultrasound" section later in this chapter for details). Between 18 and 22 weeks, you may feel the baby moving, although the movements don't necessarily occur regularly. By 26 weeks, the baby looks less like a fetus and more like a baby. The baby's head, which was large in relation to rest of its body during the first trimester, becomes more proportional. The bones solidify and are recognizable on an ultrasound.

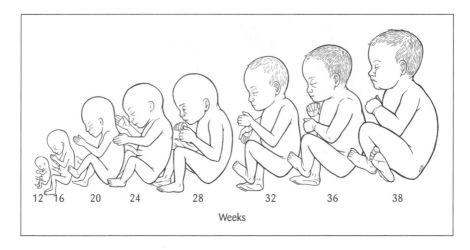

Figure 5-1: Growth during the second trimester (13–26 weeks).

The fetus performs many recognizable activities. Not only does it move, it also undergoes regular periods of sleep and wakefulness. It can hear and swallow. Lung development increases markedly between 20 and 25 weeks. By 24 weeks, lung cells begin to secrete *surfactant,* a chemical substance that enables the lungs to stay expanded. Between 26 and 28 weeks, the eyes — which had been fused shut — open. Hair, called *lanugo,* appears on the head and body. Fat deposits form under the skin. The central nervous system matures dramatically.

At 23 to 24 weeks, the fetus is considered *viable,* a medical term that means the baby has a reasonable chance of surviving if it is born at this time in a center with a neonatal unit experienced in caring for very premature babies. In fact, a premature baby born at 28 weeks, nearly three months early, that is cared for in an intensive care unit, has an excellent chance of survival.

Fetal Movements

Many women sense fluttering movements called *quickening* at about 16 to 20 weeks. Sometimes, this sensation is the baby moving, and sometimes, it's just gas. Around 20 to 22 weeks, the fetal movements are much easier to identify but still aren't consistent. In the four weeks after that, however,

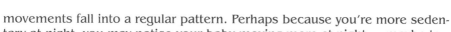
movements fall into a regular pattern. Perhaps because you're more seden-tary at night, you may notice your baby moving more at night — maybe to prepare you for the sleepless nights you'll have after she or he is born!

If you haven't felt your baby move at all by 22 weeks, let your practitioner know. He or she may recommend an ultrasound (see the "Ultrasound" sec-tion later in this chapter) to check the baby's health, especially if you haven't had an ultrasound already. Sometimes the placenta is implanted on the *anterior,* or front, wall of the uterus between the baby and your skin, and the placenta acts as a cushion that prevents you from feeling the baby move.

If you stop feeling the baby move as much as usual after 26 to 28 weeks, call your practitioner. By 28 weeks, you should feel movement at least six times an hour after you eat dinner. If you are not sure whether the baby is moving normally, lie down on your left side and count the movements.

Your Changing Body

Your body goes through many changes in the second trimester. As your baby develops inside you, your body adopts to being pregnant. You may experience some, none, or all of these symptoms (lucky you!):

* **Forgetfulness and clumsiness:** Believe it — misplacing keys, bumping into furniture, and dropping items are genuine side effects of pregnancy. If it happens to you, don't worry. You're not losing your mind; instead, you have a good excuse for being forgetful.

* **Gas:** You may develop an annoying and embarrassing tendency to burp and pass gas at inopportune times. You can do very little about it (besides getting a dog to blame it on) besides avoiding large meals and foods that make the problem worse.

* **Hair and nail growth:** Fingernails and toenails may become stronger than they've ever been before and grow at an unprece-dented rate. Pregnancy speeds up hair growth and sometimes makes hair grow in unusual places — on your face or stomach, for example. Waxing, plucking, and shaving unwanted hair is safe, but hair removal creams (depilatories) contain chemicals that have not been extensively studied, so you probably want to avoid them.

* **Heartburn:** The burning sensation you feel when stomach acid rises into your esophagus is common during pregnancy. You get heartburn because high levels of progesterone produced in your body slow digestion and relax the sphincter muscle between the esophagus and stomach that normally prevents the upward movement of acids. You also get it because, as the uterus grows, it presses upward on the stomach and pushes acid into the esophagus. If your heartburn

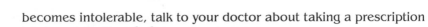
becomes intolerable, talk to your doctor about taking a prescription treatment that's safe for pregnant women.

* **Lower abdominal/groin pain:** Between 18 and 24 weeks, you may feel a sharp pain or a dull ache near or on both sides of your groin. The ache is often worse when you stand or move quickly. It may fade when you lie down. This pain is called *round ligament pain,* and, although it can be quite uncomfortable, it's normal. The round ligaments are bands of fibrous tissue on each side of the uterus that attach the top of the uterus to the labia, the lips of the external genitalia. The pain occurs because the ligaments stretch as the uterus grows.

* **Nasal congestion:** The increased blood flow that occurs during pregnancy can cause stuffiness and swelling of the mucous membranes inside your nose. This symptom, in turn, can lead to postnasal drip and, ultimately, a chronic cough, not to mention loud snoring. Nasal saline drops may provide relief and are perfectly safe during pregnancy

* **Nosebleeds and bleeding gums:** Due to the higher volume of blood coursing through your body, you may experience some bleeding from small blood vessels in your nose and gums. This bleeding usually stops on its own, but you can help by applying slight pressure to the point of bleeding. If bleeding becomes particularly heavy or frequent, call your doctor.

In addition, you may experience skin changes throughout your pregnancy. The following list outlines common changes to the skin. Don't worry. These skin changes fade away or disappear after pregnancy:

* **Linea nigra:** You may notice a dark line, called the *linea nigra,* on your lower abdomen running from your pubic bone up to your navel. This line is usually more noticeable in women with dark skin. Fair-skinned women often don't develop this line.

* **Mask of pregnancy:** The skin on your face may darken and form a masklike distribution around your cheeks, nose, and eyes. This darkening is called *chloasma* or the *mask of pregnancy.* These skin changes are caused by hormonal influences on skin pigment cells. Rest assured that this new coloring usually fades away after the baby is born.

* **Red spots:** Red spots, called *spider angiomas,* may suddenly appear anywhere on your body. Press on them, and they usually turn white. These spots are concentrations of blood vessels caused by the high level of estrogen in your body.

* **Palmar erythema:** Some women notice a reddish coloring on the palms of their hands. Known as *palmar erythema,* this coloring is another estrogen effect.

☺ ☺ ☹ ☺ ☺ ☹ ☺ ☺ ☹ ☺ ☺ ☹ ☺ ☺ ☹ ☺ ☺ ☹ ☺

❀ **Skin tags:** For reasons that are unclear, *skin tags* — small, benign skin grows — are also a common occurrence. Because they, too, disappear after pregnancy, don't rush to the dermatologist to have them removed, unless they are especially bothersome.

What to Expect at Prenatal Visits

In the second trimester, you see your practitioner roughly once every four weeks. At each visit, he or she checks your weight, your blood pressure, your urine, and the fetal heart rate. At these visits, be sure to bring up any questions you have about fetal movement, childbirth classes, your weight gain, and any unusual symptoms or discomforts.

 Your practitioner routinely performs a number of tests during the second trimester to find out whether you are at risk for such complications as diabetes, anemia, or birth defects. Sometimes, you're given an ultrasound exam so that your practitioner can find out whether you're having twins, your baby is growing normally, and you have plenty of amniotic fluid.

Second-trimester blood tests

The following blood tests are usually performed during the second trimester. Ideally, the tests show normal results right away, but if your practitioner notices anything unusual, you may need further testing — an ultrasound examination, perhaps. Remember that further testing does not necessarily mean that anything is wrong. Your practitioner is simply being careful to ensure that everything is okay.

❀ **Alpha-fetoprotein screen:** *Maternal serum alpha-fetoprotein* (MSAFP) is a protein made by the fetus that circulates in the mother's bloodstream. Between 15 and 18 weeks, doctors use a simple blood test to check for elevated MSAFP levels. Most women with an elevated MSAFP have a normal fetus and continue to have a completely normal pregnancy, but, among other things, an elevated MSAFP may indicate the presence of neural tube defects, abdominal wall defects, or that the fetus's age was underestimated.

❀ **The double, triple, and now quadruple Down syndrome screen:** Doctors also conduct a simple blood test to screen for Down syndrome, the most common chromosome abnormality in babies. This test can also help to identify women at risk of having babies with other chromosomal abnormalities, such as Trisomy 18 or Trisomy 13 (an extra copy of either the number 18 or 13 chromosome).

☺ ☺ ☹ ☺ ☺ ☹ ☺ ☺ ☹ ☺ ☺ ☹ ☺ ☺ ☹ ☺ ☺ ☺ ☹ ☺

❋ **Glucose screens:** The glucose screen helps identify women who may have gestational diabetes. In the test, you drink a nasty-tasting glucose mixture, and, exactly one hour later, a blood sample is taken. This sample is checked for the level of *glucose,* also known as *blood sugar.* High levels indicate that you are at risk for gestational diabetes.

❋ **Complete blood count (CBC):** Many obstetricians take a complete blood count at the same time that they do the glucose test in order to see whether you've developed significant anemia (iron deficiency) or a variety of other less common problems. Anemia is common during pregnancy, and some women need to take extra iron.

Ultrasound

An ultrasound exam, also called a *sonogram,* is an incredibly useful tool that allows you and your doctor to see the baby inside your uterus. An ultrasound exam doesn't hurt. The technology is safe and has been in use for more than 30 years. In the exam, a gel or lotion is spread over the abdomen. Then a device called a *transducer* that emits sound waves is moved through the gel, as shown in Figure 5-2. The sound waves are reflected off the fetus and converted into an image that appears on a monitor. You can see almost all the structures in the fetus's body. You can also see the fetus moving around and performing all its normal activities — kicking, waving, and so on. The picture quality varies, depending on maternal fat, scar tissue, and the position of the fetus. The best time to view the baby's anatomy is around 18 to 22 weeks.

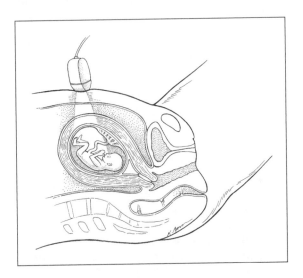

Figure 5-2: An second trimester ultrasound test.

☺ ☹ ☺ ☺ ☹ ☺ ☺ ☹ ☺ ☺ ☹ ☺ ☺ ☹ ☺ ☺ ☹ ☺

An ultrasound is like a checkup for the fetus. It can provide information about the following:

- Number of babies

- Gestational age

- Rate of fetal growth

- Fetal position, movement, and breathing exercises (the fetus moves its chest and abdomen as if it were breathing air)

- Fetal heart rate

- Amount of amniotic fluid

- Location of placenta

- Fetal anatomy, including the identification of some birth defects

- The baby's gender (after 15 to 16 weeks), although this is not always possible to see

Although ultrasound has truly revolutionized obstetrics, providing invaluable help in identifying, managing, and sometimes even treating certain problems, it isn't perfect. It can detect only half of all birth defects. It can't always identify fetuses with chromosomal abnormalities. For example, an ultrasound can detect only about half of all cases of Down syndrome in women at risk for this problem.

Amniocentesis

The purpose of amniocentesis is to check fetal chromosomes to see that 23 chromosome pairs are present and that their structure is normal, although, later in the pregnancy, the procedure may be done for other reasons, such as checking for lung maturity in the baby. Usually, the test is done at 15 to 20 weeks. With an ultrasound image of the fetus and the amniotic sac showing on the ultrasound screen, a thin, hollow needle is inserted through your abdomen, into the amniotic sac, and some amniotic fluid is withdrawn (usually about 15 to 20 cc, or 1 to 2 tablespoons), as shown in Figure 5-3. The procedure typically lasts no longer than one or two minutes, although it can seem an eternity if you are anxious. For a genetic amniocentesis, the amniotic fluid cells must be incubated, which takes some time. Results are usually available in one to two weeks.

The procedure is mildly uncomfortable but not terribly painful. Many women feel a slight, brief cramping sensation as the needle goes into the uterus and then a weird pulling sensation as the fluid is withdrawn through the needle. Afterward, your doctor may advise you to rest and avoid strenuous activity and sex for one to two days.

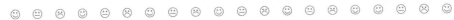

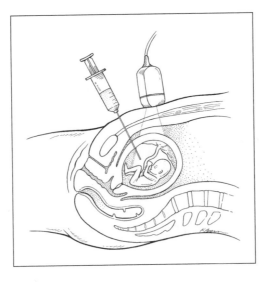

Figure 5-3: An amniocentesis procedure.

Risks and side effects of amniocentesis

Not all patients have these symptoms or problems after an amniocentesis, but it is important to be aware that they can occur.

- ❀ **Cramping:** Usually goes away within a day. The best treatment for cramping is rest. Some practitioners recommend a single glass of wine to ease the discomfort.

- ❀ **Spotting:** May last one to two days.

- ❀ **Amniotic fluid leak:** A leakage of 1 to 2 teaspoons of fluid through the vagina occurs in 1 to 2 percent of patients. In the great majority of these cases, the membrane seals over within 48 hours, leakage stops, and the pregnancy continues normally. If you experience a large amount of leakage or persistent leakage, call your doctor.

- ❀ **Fetal injury:** Injury to the fetus is extremely rare, given the use of ultrasound guidance.

- ❀ **Miscarriage:** Amniocentesis is an invasive procedure. As such, your basic risk of miscarriage goes up by percent when you have amnio-centesis. An amniocentesis done later than 20 weeks doesn't carry the same risk of miscarriage.

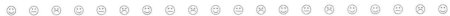

Call your doctor!

The following is a list of second-trimester symptoms that require some attention. If you experience any of them, call your practitioner.

* Bleeding

* An unusual sense of pressure or heaviness

* Regular contractions or strong cramping

* A lack of normal fetal movement

* High fever

* Severe abdominal pain

Reasons for having an amniocentesis

Genetic amniocentesis may be recommended for the following conditions or situations:

* You will be age 35 or more at your due date. This age varies from country to country and depends on the number of babies you are carrying.

* You had an elevated MSAFP (see the "Second-trimester blood tests" section earlier in this chapter).

* You had abnormal results from the Down syndrome screening.

* Your ultrasound exam was abnormal, indicating, for example, poor fetal growth or suspected structural abnormalities.

* You had a previous child or previous pregnancy with a chromosomal abnormality.

* You are at risk of having a baby with a certain genetic disease.

* You and your partner have concerns and want to confirm that the chromosomes are normal.

☺ ☺ ☹ ☺ ☺ ☹ ☺ ☺ ☹ ☺ ☺ ☹ ☺ ☺ ☹ ☺ ☺ ☺ ☹ ☺

Causes for Concern

This section discusses certain problems that can develop during the second trimester and symptoms that you should discuss with your practitioner.

❀ **Bleeding:** Some women experience bleeding in the second trimester. Possible causes include a low-lying placenta *(placenta previa)*, premature labor, cervical incompetence, or placental abruption. Sometimes no cause can be found. If you experience bleeding, it doesn't necessarily mean that you will have a miscarriage, but you should call your doctor.

❀ **Fetal abnormality:** Two to three percent of infants are born with an abnormality, and, although most of these abnormalities are minor, some lead to significant problems for the newborn. When confronted with any such situation, gather as much information as you can so that you know what to expect.

❀ **Incompetent cervix:** During the second trimester, usually between 16 and 24 weeks, some women develop a problem known as an *incompetent cervix.* The cervix opens up and dilates, even though the women feel no contractions. This condition may lead to miscarriage. In cases in which an incompetent cervix is diagnosed before the pregnancy is lost, the woman's cervix can be held shut with a stitch, called a *cerclage*, around the cervix.

Chapter 6

Not Long Now: The Third Trimester

Now you're finally ready for the third act, the final trimester of your pregnancy. By now, you're probably accustomed to your protruding belly, your morning sickness is long gone, and you've come to expect and enjoy the feeling of a baby moving around and kicking inside you. In this trimester, your baby continues to grow, and your practitioner monitors your health and your baby's health more closely than ever. You begin making preparations for the new arrival, which may mean anything from getting ready to take a leave of absence from your job to taking childbirth classes.

This chapter explores what to expect from the baby inside you, how your body changes, what to look for in prenatal visits in the third trimester, whether to take a childbirth classes, and when to alert your doctor as your delivery date approaches.

Your Baby Gets Ready for Birth

Consider how much your baby grows in the third trimester:

❀ At 28 weeks, the start of the third trimester, your baby measures about 14 inches (about 35 cm); your baby weighs about 2¹/₂ pounds (about 1,135 grams).

❀ At 40 weeks, roughly the end of the third trimester, your baby measures about 20 inches (50 cm) and weighs 6 to 8 pounds (about 2,700 to 3,600 grams) — sometimes a bit more, sometimes a bit less.

The fetus spends most of the third trimester growing, adding fat, and continuing to develop various organs, especially the central nervous system. The arms and legs get chubbier. The skin turns bluish-pink and smooth. Your fetus is less susceptible to infections and to the adverse effects of medications, although some of these agents may still affect his or her growth. The fetus spends the last two months getting ready for the transition to life in the world outside the uterus. The changes are less dramatic than they were early on, but the maturation and growth that happen now are very important.

By 28 to 34 weeks, the fetus usually assumes a head-down position, called a *vertex presentation,* as shown in Figure 6-1. In this position, the bulkiest parts of the body, the buttocks and legs, occupy the roomiest part of the uterus, the top part. In about 4 to 6 percent of single-baby pregnancies, the baby may be positioned in the *breech position,* buttocks-down, or lie across the uterus, known as the *transverse position.*

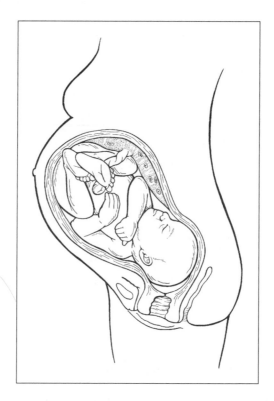

Figure 6-1: How your baby may look inside your uterus during the third trimester.

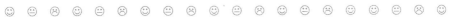

What to name your baby?

By now, you must have been asked at least once, "What are you going to name the baby?" Choosing the name that your baby will carry around for the rest of his or her life is an important decision, and one that usually involves coming to some kind of compromise with your partner. As you negotiate, keep track of your choices here and also pick up a copy of *The Parent's Success Guide to Baby Names*, edited by P. Mourouzis (Wiley).

Girl's Names	Boy's Names

By 36 weeks, growth slows, and amniotic fluid volume is at its maximum level. After this point, the amount of amniotic fluid may start to decline. In fact, most practitioners routinely check the amniotic fluid volume on ultrasound or by feeling your abdomen during the last few weeks to make sure that a normal amount remains. (See Chapter 5 for the lowdown on ultrasound exams.)

Your practitioner keeps an eye on your baby's growth rate, most often by measuring fundal height (see Chapter 2) and paying attention to your weight gain. If you've put on too little or too much weight, if your fundal height measurements are abnormal, or if something in your history puts you at risk for growth problems, your doctor is likely to send you for an ultrasound exam to more accurately assess the situation.

Fetal movements

You may feel as if a volcano is erupting inside your uterus in the third trimester. Toward the end of pregnancy, fetal movements feel less like jabs and more like tumbles or rolls. The fetus is adapting a more newborn-like

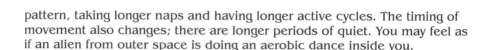

pattern, taking longer naps and having longer active cycles. The timing of movement also changes; there are longer periods of quiet. You may feel as if an alien from outer space is doing an aerobic dance inside you.

As a general rule, you should feel about six movements in the hour after dinner, while resting. Any movement, no matter how subtle, counts. Some women go for periods of feeling less fetal movement, but then the movements pick up again and are normal. This pattern is common and is not a cause for concern. However, if you notice a pattern of diminishing fetal movements or you feel absolutely no fetal movements over several hours (despite resting or eating), give your practitioner a call right away.

Breathing movements

Fetuses undergo what are called *rhythmic breathing movements* from 10 weeks onward. These movements are much more frequent in the third trimester. The fetus doesn't actually breathe. Its chest, abdominal wall, and diaphragm move in a pattern that is characteristic of breathing. You can't detect these movements, but they can be observed with ultrasound and are a sign that the baby is faring well. During the third trimester, the amount of time a fetus spends in rhythmic breathing movements increases, especially after meals.

Fetal hiccups

At times, you may feel a quick, rhythmic pattern of fetal movements occurring every few seconds. These movements are most likely hiccups. Some women feel fetal hiccups several times throughout the day; others rarely feel them. These hiccups often continue after the baby is born and are completely normal.

Keeping Up with Your Changing Body

As the baby grows, so does your belly! And, while big is beautiful, it can become uncomfortable. For example, your uterus pushes up on your ribs, which can be quite uncomfortable. Sometimes you notice kicking in one particular spot, probably where the baby's extremities are. Moving around like you used to becomes more and more difficult.

 If you find it difficult to rise from lying on your back and no one is around to help, try turning on your side first and then pushing yourself up to a sitting position.

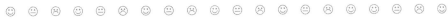

A pregnant woman knows no strangers

A pregnant woman's belly is public property. Perfect strangers put their hands on your abdomen and tell you how pleased they are that you're having a baby! Some women find this kind of attention caring and supportive; others find it annoying, embarrassing, and uncomfortable.

Many people think it perfectly polite to comment on your appearance. They tell you that you look too fat or too thin; that you are carrying too wide or all in your buttocks. They say that this or that is a sign that the baby is a boy or a girl. "Whoa, you must be about ready to pop!" they may exclaim, or "My goodness, you're enormous!" Try, if you can, *not* to pay attention to what they say. Indeed, the very best advice is not to let other people drive you crazy. They have the best of intentions, but they don't realize how their words sound to you.

Accidents and falls

If you do fall, don't worry. Chances are good that the baby remains well protected inside your uterus and its sac of amniotic fluid, which make for an excellent natural cushion. However, if you suffer severe abdominal pain, contractions, bleeding, or leakage of amniotic fluid, or if you notice a decrease in fetal movements, call your practitioner immediately. If the fall or injury involves a direct blow to your uterus, your practitioner will probably monitor your baby for a while to make sure everything is okay.

Braxton-Hicks contractions

In the late second trimester or beginning of the third trimester, your uterus may from time to time become momentarily hard or feel as though it is balling up. This feeling occurs because you're experiencing *Braxton-Hicks contractions.* They're not the kind of contractions you have in labor; they're more like practice ones.

Braxton-Hicks contractions are usually painless, but they can make you uncomfortable. They usually occur more frequently when you're active. Women who have already had children tend to notice more Braxton-Hicks contractions. You may have a hard time distinguishing Braxton-Hicks contractions from fetal movements, especially if this is your first pregnancy. Other times, Braxton-Hicks contractions can become uncomfortable and lead to false labor.

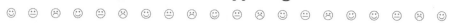
 If you are less than 36 weeks along and you experience contractions that are persistent, regular, and increasingly painful, call your doctor to make sure that you're not in premature labor.

Carpal tunnel syndrome

If you feel numbness, tingling, or pain in the fingers and wrist of one or both hands, you're probably experiencing *carpal tunnel syndrome.* It occurs when swelling in the wrist puts pressure on the *median nerve,* the nerve that runs through the *carpal tunnel* from the wrist to the hand. The pain may be worse at night or upon awakening.

If carpal tunnel syndrome becomes persistent or bothersome, discuss it with your practitioner. Wrist splints, available at some drug stores and surgical supply stores, can relieve the problem. Try not to be discouraged if it doesn't seem to get better, because it usually improves, often dramatically, after delivery.

Dropping or lightening

During the month before delivery, your belly may drop lower, and your breathing may come more easily. If you have heartburn, it improves. These symptoms happen because the baby has *dropped,* or *lightened* — in other words, descended lower into the pelvis. Typically, it happens two to three weeks before delivery if you're having your first child (women who have had children before may not drop until they are in labor). Your uterus doesn't press up on your diaphragm or stomach as much as it used to, so breathing is easier, and heartburn improves. At the same time, however, you may feel more pressure in your vaginal area. Some women report feeling strange, sharp twinges as the baby's head moves and exerts pressure on the bladder and pelvic floor.

Some women don't notice that they've dropped. During your prenatal visit, your doctor may undertake an external or internal exam to see how low the baby's head is and whether it's engaged. As shown in Figure 6-2, *engaged* means that the fetal head has reached the level of the *ischial spines,* the bony landmarks in your pelvis that can be felt during an internal exam.

When the fetal head is at this level, it is said to be at *zero station.* Most practitioners divide the pelvis into descending stations from –5 to +5 (some use a scale of –3 to +3). Often at the beginning of labor, the head is at –4 or –5 station. In this position — sometimes called *floating* — it is considered fairly high, because the fetal head is still floating in the amniotic cavity. Labor proceeds when the head descends all the way to +5, and delivery is about to begin.

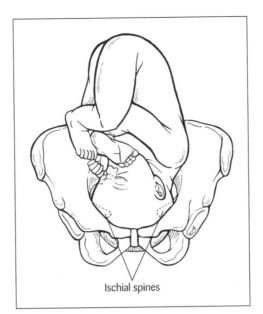

Figure 6-2: This baby is said to be engaged.

If the baby's head is engaged prior to labor, you're more likely to deliver vaginally. While a floating (unengaged) head isn't every obstetrician's dream, it doesn't mean that you won't have a completely normal delivery. If you're having your second child or more, the baby's head may not engage until well into labor.

Fatigue

The fatigue you felt early in your pregnancy may return in the third trimester. You may feel as if you're slowing down. Much of the time, you're tired, you're carrying around more weight, and you're uncomfortable. Often, the second or third pregnancy is more tiring than the first because you now have older children to care for.

Try to be realistic about what you can do and don't feel guilty about what you can't get done. Take time for yourself and get as much rest as you can. Delegate tasks. Whenever possible, let other people help with household chores and other responsibilities. Do whatever you can to take advantage of the quiet times. Rest as much as you can now, because after delivery, the work really picks up!

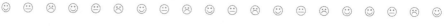

Hemorrhoids

No one wants to talk about them, but *hemorrhoids* — dilated, swollen veins around the rectum — are a common problem for pregnant women. Hemorrhoids are essentially varicose veins of the rectum (see the "Varicose veins" section later in this chapter). They're caused by the uterus pressing on major blood vessels, which leads to pooling of blood, and ultimately makes the veins enlarge and swell. Progesterone relaxes the veins, allowing the swelling to increase. Constipation makes hemorrhoids worse. Straining and pushing hard during bowel movements puts added pressure on the blood vessels, causing them to enlarge and possibly protrude from the rectum.

Hemorrhoids sometimes bleed. This bleeding doesn't harm the pregnancy, but if it becomes frequent, talk to your doctor about seeing a colorectal specialist. If hemorrhoids become very painful, you may want to discuss whether treatment is necessary. Meanwhile, you can try the following:

- **Avoid constipation** (see Chapter 4).

- **Exercise.**

- **Get off your feet when you can.** Doing so alleviates extra pressure on your veins.

- **Try over-the-counter topical medications such as Preparation H or Anusol.**

- **Take warm baths two to three times a day.** Soaking in warm (not hot!) water can help relieve the muscle spasms that most often cause the pain.

- **Use over-the-counter hemorrhoidal pads (such as Tucks) or witch hazel pads to clean and medicate the area.**

Pushing during the second stage of labor (see Chapter 7) can make hemorrhoids worse or make them appear where they were not before. But most of the time, hemorrhoids go away after delivery.

Insomnia

During the last few months of pregnancy, many women find sleeping quite difficult. The fact is, finding a comfortable position when you're eight months along is difficult. You feel a little like a beached whale. Getting up five times a night to go to the bathroom doesn't make things any easier. However, you may find relief in the following:

- **Drink warm milk with honey.** Warming the milk releases *tryptophan*, a naturally occurring amino acid that makes you sleepy; the honey causes you to produce insulin, which also makes you drowsy.

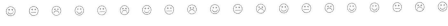

- **Get in some exercise during the day.**

- **Go to bed a little later than usual.**

- **Limit your liquid intake after 6 p.m.** Don't limit it to the point that you become dehydrated, however.

- **Invest in a body pillow.** You can tuck it around your body in various places, helping you find a comfortable position. You can get a body pillow in almost any department store.

- **Take a warm, relaxing bath before going to bed.**

Pregnancy rashes and itches

Pregnant women are subject to the same rashes that non-pregnant women get. *Pruritic urticarial papules of pregnancy,* or PUPP, however, is unique to pregnancy. This rash is more of a nuisance than anything else, and it can cause intense itching. PUPP tends to occur late in pregnancy and is characterized by hives or red patches that first appear in the stretch marks on your abdomen. These patches can spread to other areas on the abdomen and to the legs, arms, chest, and back. They almost never spread to the face (thank heaven for small favors). The good news is that the condition poses no risk to the baby, although your doctor may recommend blood tests to make sure you don't have other conditions that are associated with itching. The only surefire way to make PUPP go away is to deliver.

Even if you don't have a rash, you may itch a lot, especially over your belly. Itching is common and usually is caused by the stretching of your skin as the baby gets bigger. It often itches most where stretch marks develop.

Sciatica

Some women experience pain extending from their lower back to their buttocks and down one leg or the other. This pain or, less commonly, numbness, is known as *sciatica.* Sciatica is caused by pressure on the sciatic nerve, a major nerve that branches from your back, through your pelvis, to your hips, and down your legs. Mild cases of sciatica can be relieved by bed rest (shift from side to side to find the position that's most comfortable), warm (not hot) baths, or heating pads applied to the painful areas. If you develop a severe case of sciatica, you may need prolonged bed rest or special exercises. Ask your doctor.

Shortness of breath

As pregnancy proceeds, you may become increasingly short of breath. The hormone progesterone affects your central breathing center and may

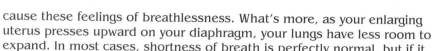
cause these feelings of breathlessness. What's more, as your enlarging uterus presses upward on your diaphragm, your lungs have less room to expand. In most cases, shortness of breath is perfectly normal, but if it comes on very suddenly or if it comes with chest pain, call your doctor.

Stretch marks

Stretch marks are an almost inevitable part of pregnancy. They are caused by the skin stretching to accommodate the enlarging uterus and the weight gain. Some women have a genetic predisposition for stretch marks. The marks typically appear as pinkish-red streaks along the abdomen and breasts, and they fade to silvery gray or white several months after delivery. Their exact color depends on your skin tone.

No cream or ointment is completely effective in preventing stretch marks. Many people think that rubbing vitamin E oil on the belly helps prevent stretch marks or helps them fade faster, but the effectiveness of vitamin E has never been proven scientifically. Women have used numerous concoctions to avoid stretch marks, but none of these products works for all women. Your best bet is to avoid excessive weight gain and to exercise regularly to maintain muscle tone, thus easing the pressure of the uterus on the overlying skin.

Swelling (edema)

Swelling of the hands and legs, called *edema*, is common in the third trimester. It usually occurs after you've been on your feet for a while, but it can occur throughout the day. Swelling tends to occur more often when the weather is warm.

 Although swelling is a normal symptom of pregnancy, it can occasionally be a sign of preeclampsia (see the "Preeclampsia" section later in this chapter for details). If you notice a sudden increase in the amount of swelling; or a sudden, large weight gain — 5 pounds or more in a week; or if the swelling is associated with significant headache or right-sided abdominal pain, call your practitioner immediately.

Contrary to myth, no evidence indicates that lowering your salt intake prevents swelling or makes it go away. For ordinary swelling, try the following:

- **Keep your legs elevated whenever possible.**
- **Stay in a cool environment.** In summer, avoid spending prolonged periods of time in the hot weather.

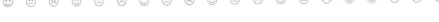

* Wear supportive pantyhose or stockings, but nothing that's too tight around your knees.

* When in bed, don't lie flat on your back; try to lie on your side.

Urinary stress incontinence

Leaking a little urine when you cough, laugh, or sneeze isn't unusual when you're pregnant. *Urinary stress incontinence* occurs because your growing uterus is putting pressure on your bladder. Relaxation of the pelvic floor muscles increases the problem during the late second and third trimesters. And sometimes, the baby gives the bladder a swift kick and causes it to leak urine.

Kegel exercises — in which you repeatedly contract the pelvic floor muscles as if you're trying very hard not to urinate — can prevent or markedly reduce this problem. Some women continue to experience a little stress incontinence even after delivery, but it usually goes away after 6 to 12 months. If you had a particularly difficult labor, where you pushed for a long time, or you had a very large baby, stress incontinence may not completely go away. Give yourself a least six months to see whether it goes away, and if it doesn't go away, talk to your doctor about how to proceed.

Varicose veins

You may notice a small road map suddenly appearing on your lower legs (and sometimes the vulvar area). These marks are dilated veins, or *varicose veins.* They are caused by the pressure of the uterus on major blood vessels, particularly the *inferior vena cava,* the vein that returns blood to the heart, and the pelvic veins. Adding to the problem, pregnancy causes the muscle tissue inside your veins to relax and your blood volume to increase. Women with light skin or with a family history of varicose veins are particularly susceptible.

Very often, the bluish-purple highways fade after delivery, but sometimes they do not disappear completely. They are painless for the most part, but occasionally may be associated with discomfort, aches, or pain. In rare instances, a blood clot develops in the superficial veins of the legs and leads to superficial thrombophlebitis. This is not a serious problem and can be treated with rest, leg elevation, warm compresses, and sometimes special stockings.

☺ ☹ ☺ ☺ ☺ ☹ ☺ ☺ ☹ ☺ ☺ ☹ ☺ ☺ ☹ ☺ ☺ ☺ ☹ ☺

You can't prevent getting varicose veins (you can't fight heredity), but you may be able to reduce their number and severity by following these tips:

✿ **Avoid standing for prolonged periods of time.**

✿ **Avoid wearing clothes that are very tight around one part of your leg.**

✿ **If you must be stationary, move your legs around from time to time to stimulate circulation.**

✿ **Keep your legs elevated whenever you can.**

✿ **Wear support stockings or talk to your doctor about a prescription for special elastic stockings.**

The Home Stretch: Prenatal Visits in the Third Trimester

Chapters 4 and 5 describe tests that are given to pregnant women in the first and second trimester. The good news is that far fewer tests are administered in the third trimester. However, between 28 and 36 weeks, your doctor probably wants to see you more frequently. Prenatal visits occur every two to three weeks and then weekly as you close in on delivery. The usual measurements are taken: blood pressure, weight, fetal heart rate, fundal height (see Chapter 2), and urine tests. Typically, Group B strep cultures are taken, and, in some instances, amniocentesis for lung maturity is performed, too; both are discussed in this section, as are a few other tests.

Group B strep cultures

The only routine test that may be performed during a third-trimester prenatal visit is a culture for *Group B strep,* a bacteria commonly found in the vagina and rectum. Within the scientific community, doctors argue over whether women should be routinely screened for Group B strep. Some obstetricians perform this test at 36 weeks; others don't. Fifteen to 20 percent of women harbor Group B strep. If the culture is positive at 36 weeks, your doctor may recommend taking antibiotics during labor to reduce the risk of transmitting the bacteria to the baby. Treating this bacteria any earlier doesn't help, because it can come back by the time you're in labor. Currently, no tests that yield immediate results are available. Because you can't test for Group B strep at the time of labor, it must be done in advance.

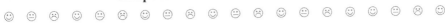

"When am I going to have my baby?"

"When am I going to have this baby?" is a question every pregnant woman asks as the end approaches. Sometimes, a woman whose cervix is long and closed goes into labor within 12 hours of an internal exam. Other women walk around with a cervix dilated to 3 centimeters for weeks! Signs that labor is near include loss of the *mucous plug* (not really a plug but thick mucous produced in the cervix), *bloody show* (a blood-tinged mucous discharge), increasing frequency of Braxton-Hicks contractions, and diarrhea. But nothing is a sure sign. Loss of the mucous plug or bloody show may occur hours, days, or weeks before labor, or in some cases, not at all.

Amniocentesis for lung maturity

If you're planning a repeat cesarean delivery (you had one in an earlier pregnancy) or you plan to induce delivery at less than 39 weeks, practitioners currently recommend having an amniocentesis to make sure that the fetus's lungs are mature and ready to function. Chapter 5 describes amniocentesis.

Testing the fetus's health

At certain times, your practitioner may suggest undergoing tests for the baby. These tests, also referred to as *antepartum fetal surveillance,* are designed to check the baby's well-being. The tests can be performed at any time after about 24 to 26 weeks if cause for concern exists, or after 41 weeks if delivery has not yet occurred. Here are the *antepartum fetal surveillance* tests:

- **Non-stress test (NST):** Non-stress testing consists of measuring the fetal heart rate, fetal movement, and uterine activity by a special monitoring machine. The doctor then looks at the tracing for signs of *accelerations,* or increases, in the fetal heart rate.

- **Contraction stress test (CST):** The contraction stress test is similar to a non-stress test except that the fetal heart is timed in relation to uterine contractions.

- **Biophysical profile (BPP):** Using ultrasound, the biophysical profile evaluates fetal movements, fetal body tone, fetal breathing movements, and the quantity of amniotic fluid.

☺ ☻ ☹ ☺ ☺ ☹ ☺ ☺ ☹ ☺ ☺ ☹ ☺ ☺ ☹ ☺ ☺ ☺ ☺ ☹ ☺

❀ **Vibracoustic stimulation:** A vibracoustic stimulation test may be performed during a non-stress test, but the fetus's response to stimulation by sound or vibrations is observed. The practitioner "buzzes" the mother's belly with a vibrating device, which causes a transmission of sound or vibrations to the fetus. Normally, the fetal heart rate accelerates when the fetus is stimulated in this way.

❀ **Doppler velocimetry:** A Doppler velocimetry test is done only in certain situations, for example, if certain fetal problems such as intrauterine growth restriction exist, or if you have high blood pressure.

❀ **Fetal kick counts:** Fetal kick counting is a way for you to test for fetal well-being at home. Lie down on your left side after dinner and count fetal movements. You should feel at least six movements within one hour.

Causes for Concern

During the final weeks and months of pregnancy, you see your practitioner more often than before. Still, certain questions and problems may arise between visits. The following sections discuss concerns that are worth alerting a doctor about.

Bleeding

If you experience significant bleeding, let your practitioner know immediately. Some third-trimester bleeding is harmless to you and your baby, but some can have serious implications. Possible causes of third-trimester bleeding include preterm labor, inflammation of the cervix, placenta previa, and placental separation.

Breech presentation

A baby is in a so-called *breech* position when its buttocks or legs are down, closest to the cervix. Breech presentation happens in 3 to 4 percent of all single-baby deliveries. A woman's risk of having a breech baby decreases the further along she goes in her pregnancy. Many practitioners recommend that all breech babies be delivered by cesarean section, but many fetuses in breech position are actually good candidates for vaginal delivery.

If you and your practitioner decide that a vaginal breech delivery is not right for you, another option is *external cephalic version,* a procedure in which the doctor tries to turn the baby into normal delivery position by externally manipulating the mother's abdomen. This is a common procedure and is usually safe.

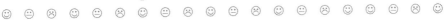

Decreased amniotic fluid volume

The medical term for decreased amniotic fluid volume is *oligohydramnios* (it used to be called *dry birth*). Usually, a mild decrease in amniotic fluid is not a major cause for concern, but your practitioner monitors it closely nonetheless with non-stress tests and ultrasound exams.

Decreased fetal movement

If you're not feeling the amount of fetal movement that you've been accustomed to, let your doctor know. Fetal movement is one of the most important details to pay attention to as you near your due date (see the "Testing the fetus's health" section earlier in this chapter).

Fetal growth problems

You may be told at a routine prenatal visit that your uterus is measuring either too big or too small. This phenomenon is not a cause for immediate alarm. Often in this situation, your practitioner suggests an ultrasound exam (see Chapter 5) to get a better idea of how big the baby is.

Leaking amniotic fluid

If you notice that your underwear is wet, several explanations are possible. It may be a little urine, vaginal discharge, the release of the mucous plug in the cervix, or actual leakage of amniotic fluid (also known as *rupture of the membranes*). Often, you can tell what it is by examining the fluid. Mucous discharge tends to be thick and globby, while vaginal discharge is whitish and smooth. Urine has its characteristic odor and isn't continuous. Amniotic fluid, on the other hand, is normally clear and watery and often is lost in spurts.

If you leak what you think is amniotic fluid, call your practitioner right away. If you're not *preterm* — if you're less than 37 weeks along — and the amniotic fluid is clear, leaking fluid is not an emergency, but most practitioners want you to call them so they can tell you what to do.

Macrosomia

Although a big, healthy, chubby baby is beautiful and wonderful, you can get too much of a good thing. A fetus is considered *macrosomic*, exceptionally large, if it weighs in above the 90th percentile or it weighs at least 8 pounds, 13 ounces (4,000 grams). Macrosomia can mean extra long labor, may put a woman at risk of needing a cesarean delivery, and increases the chance of having a difficult delivery.

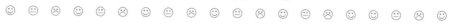

Preeclampsia

Preeclampsia, in which high blood pressure is associated with the spilling of protein into the urine and sometimes swelling *(edema)* in the hands, face, and legs, is a condition unique to pregnancy. Preeclampsia, also called *toxemia* or *pregnancy-induced hypertension,* isn't uncommon. It occurs in 6 to 8 percent of all pregnancies. It can be very mild or be a serious medical condition.

Preterm labor

The strict technical definition of preterm labor is when a woman begins to have contractions and changes in her cervix before she is 37 weeks along. Many women have contractions but no cervical change, in which case, it isn't real preterm labor. However, in order to find out whether your cervix is changing, you need to be examined. Your practitioner determines how often you are contracting by placing you on a uterine contraction monitor similar to the one used to perform a non-stress test (see the "Testing the fetus's health" section earlier in this chapter). If labor occurs after 35 weeks, your practitioner probably won't try to stop your contractions except in rare circumstances, such as poorly controlled diabetes.

When the baby is late

For nearly nine months, you believe that your baby is coming on a certain date, your due date. The fact is, though, that only about 5 percent of women actually deliver on their due date. Eighty percent deliver between 37 and 42 weeks, which is considered full term. Ten percent don't deliver by 42 weeks. These prolonged pregnancies are known as *post-date* or *post-term* pregnancies. At one time, these pregnancies were often the result of incorrectly estimated due dates, but today, with the widespread use of ultrasound, due dates are pretty accurate.

Many practitioners advise that labor be induced if the pregnancy reaches 42 weeks. If it goes on any longer, the baby is likely to still be fine, but greater health risks are possible.

Going Back to School: Taking a Childbirth Class

Today's birthing experience is a far cry from earlier in this century, when women were knocked out with anesthesia for the delivery, and the expectant father's only job was to pace around the waiting room like Ricky Ricardo anticipating the arrival of Little Ricky. Today, a great majority of first-time expectant parents attend childbirth classes. The parents-to-be

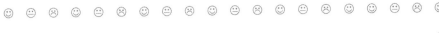
find out what experiences to anticipate and meet other expectant parents. They also find out about techniques — such as breathing, relaxation, and massage — to alleviate the fear, anxiety, and even the pain associated with labor. The greatest benefit of childbirth classes is probably the opportunity they provide to find out what to anticipate during labor, because a little information goes a long way in reducing anxiety and fear about the big event.

If you decide to take a class, make sure that the one you choose provides reliable and accurate information. Ask your practitioner for recommendations or ask friends who have already attended classes. A tour of the hospital or childbirth center where you plan to deliver often occurs as part of your childbirth education class. (If it doesn't, ask your practitioner about arranging a tour.)

Several methods of childbirth preparation are available. These methods are designed to help you discover how to deal with pain and to lower your anxiety and discomfort about what lies ahead:

❋ **Lamaze:** Perhaps the most well known of all the techniques, Lamaze focuses on shallow, rapid breathing to make the pain endurable. It teaches you ways to concentrate and relax by practicing planned responses to contractions. Your coach — the baby's father or other person close to you — helps you practice, and ultimately apply, the techniques.

❋ **Bradley method:** This method is a collection of techniques for deep abdominal breathing and relaxation to decrease the pain of labor. The emphasis is on developing your ability to concentrate on what's going on inside your body. Your partner participates to help you focus on your body and deal with the pain. Although the goal of this method is to enable you to deliver without anesthesia, don't feel like a failure if labor turns out to be more difficult than you expected, and you end up asking for medication.

❋ **Grantly Dick-Read:** The basic premise behind this technique is that the pain of labor results largely from the mother's fear of the unknown. Educating the patient about the childbirth process decreases that fear and its associated tension, and thereby decreases the pain of labor.

☺ ☺ ☹ ☺ ☺ ☺ ☹ ☺ ☺ ☹ ☺ ☺ ☹ ☺ ☺ ☹ ☺ ☺ ☺ ☹ ☺

Part 3

What You've Been Waiting For: The Big Day

And now, the moment you've been waiting for. . . .

Like pregnancy itself, childbirth can go more smoothly if you know what's going to happen. You can benefit by being aware, for example, of the different ways you can deliver your baby and the different choices you can make about anesthesia. This part is filled with details about childbirth, so that you can get ready for the big event.

Chapter 7

Labor Day – More Than a Sign to Stop Wearing White

Despite the incredible advances that have been made in science and medicine, no one really knows what causes labor to begin. A combination of stimuli originating in the mother, the baby, and the placenta may start labor. Rising levels of steroid-like substances in the mother or other biochemical substances produced by the baby may also bring about labor.

Most women can't be certain whether they are really in labor. Even a woman expecting her third or fourth child doesn't always know. Don't be surprised if you call your practitioner several times or make many trips to the hospital or birthing center, only to find out that you aren't really in labor.

This chapter helps you identify when you're entering labor and understand the many changes that occur in your body. You uncover the three stages of labor so that you can be better prepared every step of the way. You also find out what complications may arise and how practitioners handle these problems. Finally, this chapter gives you a great deal of information about managing pain during labor — something every expectant mother thinks about!

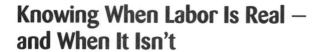

Knowing When Labor Is Real — and When It Isn't

You may experience early symptoms of labor before labor actually begins. These early labor-like symptoms are merely nature's way of suggesting that labor may occur in the next few days or weeks. Some women experience them for days or weeks; others for only a few hours. Going into labor isn't usually as dramatic as it is portrayed on sitcoms (picture Lucy saying, "Ricky, this is it!"). Women very rarely fail to make it to the hospital before they deliver.

 If you think you're in active labor, don't run to the hospital right away. Instead, telephone your practitioner first.

Noticing changes before labor begins

As you near the end of your pregnancy, you may notice some or all of these changes:

* **Bloody show:** As changes in your cervix take place, you may expel mucous discharge mixed with blood from your vagina. The blood doesn't come from your uterus, where the baby is; it comes from small, broken capillaries in your cervix.

* **Diarrhea:** Usually a few days before labor, your body releases *prostaglandins*. These substances help the uterus contract and may cause diarrhea.

* **Dropping and engagement:** Especially in women who are giving birth for the first time, the fetus often drops into the pelvis several weeks before labor (see Chapter 6 for more information). Consequently, you may feel increased pressure on your vagina and sharp pains radiating to your vagina. On the other hand, you also may notice that your whole uterus is lower in your belly and that you are suddenly more comfortable and can breathe more easily.

* **Increase in Braxton-Hicks contractions:** You may notice an increase in the frequency and strength of *Braxton-Hicks contractions* (see Chapter 6). These contractions may become somewhat uncomfortable, even if they don't grow any stronger or more frequent. Some women experience strong Braxton-Hicks contractions for weeks before labor begins.

* **Mucous discharge:** You may secrete a thick mucous discharge known as the *mucous plug*. During your pregnancy, this substance plugs your cervix, protecting your uterus from infection. As your cervix starts to thin out *(efface)* and dilate in preparation for delivery, the plug may wash out.

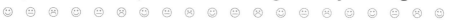
Telling the difference between false labor and true labor

Telling the difference true and false labor isn't always easy. In general, you're in false labor if your contractions are irregular and don't increase in frequency; disappear when you change position, walk, or rest; occur only in your lower abdomen; and don't become increasingly uncomfortable.

On the other hand, you're more likely to be in actual labor if your contractions grow steadily more intense and more uncomfortable; don't go away when you change position, walk, or rest; occur along with leakage of fluid (due to rupture of the membranes); make normal talking difficult or impossible; stretch across your upper abdomen or are located in your back, radiating to your front.

You are considered to be in labor if you are having regular contractions, and your cervix is changing fairly rapidly — effacing, dilating, or both. Sometimes women walk around for weeks with a partially dilated or effaced cervix but are not considered to be in labor because these changes are occurring over weeks instead of hours.

To sum up, Table 7-1 outlines the differences between true and false labor.

Table 7-1 True Versus False Labor

Characteristic	False Labor	True Labor
Contraction frequency	Irregular; no increase in frequency	Regular; contractions become closer and closer together
Contraction length	Irregular	40 to 60 seconds
Contraction intensity	No increase; not particularly uncomfortable	Grow increasingly more painful
When you change position	Contractions go away	No change, or an increase in contractions
Location of contraction	Lower abdomen	Upper abdomen or lower back, radiating to the lower abdomen

 Here's a little trick for finding out whether you're truly experiencing contractions. With your fingertips, touch your cheek and then your forehead. Finally, touch the top part of your abdomen, through which you can feel the top part of your uterus (the fundus). A relaxed uterus feels soft, like your cheek, and a contracting uterus feels hard, like your forehead.

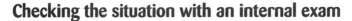
Checking the situation with an internal exam

Sometimes the only way you can know for sure whether you're in labor is by seeing your practitioner or going to the hospital. When a practitioner is trying to determine whether you're in labor, he or she performs an internal exam to look for several features:

❀ **Dilation:** Your cervix is closed for most of your pregnancy but may gradually start to dilate during the last couple of weeks, especially if you've had a baby before. Usually, you are considered to be in active labor when your cervix is about 4 centimeters dilated or 100 percent effaced.

❀ **Effacement:** Effacement is a thinning out or shortening of the cervix, which happens during labor. Your cervix goes from being thick *(uneffaced)* to 100 percent effaced.

❀ **Station:** When you're in labor, the practitioner uses the term *station* to describe how far your baby's head (or other presenting part) has descended in the birth canal in relation to the *ischial spines,* a bony landmark in your pelvis. These stations are numbered from –5 (or sometimes –3) to +5 (or +3). A station of –5 (or –3) indicates that the baby's head is at the highest point on the scale, and a station of +5 (or +3) indicates that the baby's head is at the lowest point on the scale and closest to delivery.

❀ **Position:** When labor begins, the baby typically starts out facing to the side (left or right). As labor progresses, the baby rotates until the head assumes a face-down position, so that the baby comes out looking at the floor. Occasionally, the baby rotates to the opposite position and comes out sunny-side up, looking at the ceiling.

When to call your practitioner

If you think you're in labor, call your practitioner. Don't be embarrassed if he or she tells you that you're probably *not* in labor (it happens to many women). Before you call, however, you may want to time your contractions for several hours to see whether they're getting closer together, because your practitioner can use this information to help determine whether you're in true labor. If your contractions are occurring every 5 to 10 minutes and are uncomfortable, definitely call. If you're less than 37 weeks pregnant and feeling persistent contractions, don't sit for hours counting their frequency — call your practitioner immediately.

Call your practitioner if any of the following apply to you:

❀ Your contractions are coming closer together, and they're becoming increasingly uncomfortable.

❀ You have ruptured membranes. Having your water break may come as a small amount of watery fluid leaking out, or it may be a big gush. If the fluid is green, brown, or red, let your practitioner know right away.

❀ You have heavy bleeding (more than a heavy menstrual period) or are passing clots.

❀ You are not feeling an adequate amount of fetal movement.

❀ You have constant, severe abdominal pain with no relief between contractions.

❀ You feel a fetal part or umbilical cord in your vagina. In this case, go to the hospital right away!

Use Table 7-2 to record when your contractions occur and how long they last. In the first column, enter the date and time of the contraction. In the second, record how long it lasted. The third column is for describing what the contraction felt like or recording anything else that seems important to you.

Table 7-2 Timing Your Contractions

Contraction Date/Time	Duration	Notes

Getting Admitted to the Hospital

If you're in labor, you're being induced into labor, or you're having an elective cesarean delivery, you will be admitted to the hospital's labor floor. If

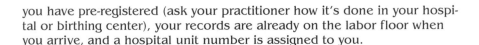
you have pre-registered (ask your practitioner how it's done in your hospital or birthing center), your records are already on the labor floor when you arrive, and a hospital unit number is assigned to you.

Some women go through labor in the same room in which they deliver the baby; others are moved to a different room for delivery. Besides the bed, the hospital room you're placed in probably includes all of the following:

- **Fetal monitor:** A machine with two attachments, one to monitor the baby's heart rate and one to monitor your contractions. The fetal monitor generates a *fetal heart tracing*, which is a paper record of how the baby's heart rate rises and falls in relation to your contractions.

- **Doppler/stethoscope:** Portable tools used for listening periodically to the fetal heartbeat, instead of using the continuous fetal monitor.

- **Infant warmer:** A heat lamp to keep the newborn's body temperature from dropping.

- **IV line:** A tube that's connected to a bag of *saline* (salt water) containing a glucose mixture to keep you properly hydrated.

Fetal Heart Monitoring

Labor puts stress on you and the baby. Fetal heart monitoring is a way to make sure the baby is handling stress. In some hospitals, all patients in labor are routinely monitored. In others, patients who are at low risk for complications are monitored intermittently. Most hospitals and most practitioners have their own ways of deciding when it's time to use fetal monitors. Sometimes, knowing whether it makes sense to use continuous monitoring isn't possible until you are in labor and your practitioner can see how the baby is responding. Monitoring is done using several techniques, including external and internal monitoring.

External monitoring

An external fetal heart monitor gives information about the fetus's response to contractions. It records *long-term variability* — that is, periodic changes in heart rate. Either two belts or a wide, elastic band are placed around the abdomen, and a device attached to the belt or band uses an ultrasound-Doppler technique to pick up the fetal heartbeat. A second device uses a gauge to pick up the contractions. An external monitor can show the frequency and duration of contractions, but it can't provide information about how strong contractions are.

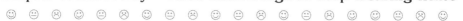

Oxytocin

Oxytocin, a synthetic hormone similar to one that your body naturally releases during labor, can be administered to induce labor. Oxytocin (brand name, Pitocin) may be used to augment labor that's already happening. If your contractions are thought to be inadequate or if labor is taking an unusually long time, your practitioner may use oxytocin to help move things along. The contractions produced as a result of this augmentation are no stronger and no more painful than contractions that occur during a spontaneous labor.

Internal monitoring

Practitioners use an internal fetal heart monitor when they need to observe the fetus more closely than they can with an external monitoring device. Practitioners use an internal fetal monitor (also called an internal scalp electrode) when they are concerned about how the fetus is tolerating labor or when they are having difficulty picking up the heart rate externally. Before a practitioner can place the internal fetal monitor, the membranes (the bag of water) must be ruptured and the cervix dilated to at least 1 or 2 centimeters. The monitor is passed through the cervix via a flexible plastic tube, and the tiny electrode is then attached to the baby's scalp. This procedure is no more uncomfortable than a pelvic exam. It is quite safe and rarely causes a local infection or a slight rash on the baby's head.

An internal monitor for contractions — called an *internal pressure transducer,* or IPT — is used to assess how strong the contractions are. Practitioners use this monitor when labor is progressing slowly in order to determine whether you require oxytocin (see the "Oxytocin" sidebar) to strengthen your contractions (see the "Inducing labor" section later in this chapter). The monitor consists of thin, flexible, fluid-filled tubing that's inserted between the fetal head and the uterine wall during an internal exam. Sometimes, this same device is used to infuse saline into the uterus — if very little amniotic fluid is present, the fetal heart tracing indicates that the umbilical cord is getting compressed or very thick *meconium* (fecal matter from the baby) is present.

Inducing Labor

To *induce* labor means to cause it to begin before it starts on its own. This section discusses the two reasons to induce and also explains how the process works.

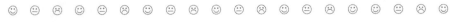
Two reasons for induction

Induction is *elective* if it is performed for the convenience of the patient or her practitioner. It is *indicated* if it is necessary on account of obstetrical, medical, or fetal complications.

Elective induction

Some practitioners gladly perform elective inductions; others are opposed to the whole concept. Here are reasons why a patient may choose to undergo an elective induction:

❀ She finds it easier to make arrangements for her other children, for her work or her partner's work, or for the convenience of other family members.

❀ She wants to ensure that a physician in a group practice with whom she has developed a special relationship delivers her baby.

❀ She is at risk for certain neonatal or labor complications and needs to deliver when the maximum number of labor floor personnel or other specialists are present.

❀ She has a history of poor pregnancy outcomes (such as a previous full-term fetal death), and she is anxious over this past experience.

❀ She lives far from the hospital and has a history of rapid deliveries.

Studies in the medical literature suggest that elective induction increases the chances of a cesarean delivery. If the cervix is neither dilated nor *effaced* (thinned out), or if the fetal head is not engaged in the pelvis, the risk of a cesarean delivery probably is higher. The length of time that a patient spends in the hospital does increase slightly when labor is induced.

Indicated induction

An induction is *indicated* when the risks of continuing the pregnancy are greater than the risks of early delivery. Problems with the mother's health that may warrant induction include preeclampsia, the presence of diseases such as diabetes or *cholestasis* (a disorder of the liver), an infection such as chorioamnionitis in the amniotic fluid, and fetal death.

Problems with the baby's health that may warrant induction include a pregnancy continuing well past the due date, ruptured membranes (which can place the baby at risk for developing an infection), intrauterine growth restriction, suspected *macrosomia* (large fetus), an Rh incompatibility with complications, decreased amniotic fluid *(oligohydramnios)*, and well-being tests that indicate that the fetus is not thriving in the uterus.

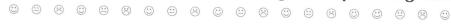
How labor is induced

How labor is induced depends upon whether your cervix is *ripe* (thinned out, soft, and dilated):

❀ If your cervix is not yet ripe, you will likely be admitted to the hospital in the evening and given medications to ripen the cervix at bedtime. Then oxytocin can be administered to induce labor in the morning.

   Various medications and techniques are used to ripen the cervix. The most common medication is a type of *prostaglandin* — a substance that helps soften cervical tissue and cause contractions — administered either as a gel or a tablet and placed in the vagina. Some practitioners prefer to use what's called a *Foley balloon,* a tiny balloon placed in the cervix through the vagina and inflated with saline or air to help the cervix open up.

❀ If your cervix is already ripe, you'll likely be admitted in the morning. Labor is induced either by administering oxytocin intravenously or by rupturing your membranes (often called *breaking your water*). An *amniotomy,* or rupturing of the membranes, is done with a small plastic hook during an internal examination. This procedure is usually not painful.

The Stages of Labor

Each woman's labor is unique. And the same woman's experience may differ from pregnancy to pregnancy. Anyone who delivers babies knows all too well that labor always surprises you. A delivery that doctors expect to go quickly takes a long time, while one doctors think will take forever sometimes goes very rapidly. Still, in the vast majority of pregnant women, labor progresses in a predictable pattern. It passes through discernible stages — the first, second, and third — at a fairly standard rate.

Practitioners can track your progress through labor by performing internal exams every few hours. How easily you progress through labor is measured by how quickly your cervix dilates and how smoothly the fetus descends downward through the pelvis and birth canal. Your practitioner may track your progress by means of a special graph called a labor curve, as shown in Figure 7-1. This graph illustrates how the labor is progressing by comparing your progress to a standard curve representing the average labor.

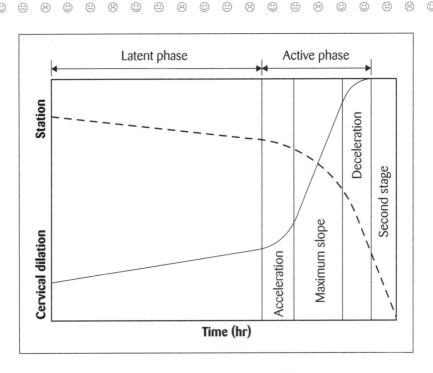

Figure 7-1: Your practitioner may use a labor curve.

If you're going through your first delivery (that is, you are what's known as a *nullipara*), the entire labor process is likely to last between 12 and 14 hours. For deliveries after the first one (for *multiparas*), labor is usually shorter, at about 8 hours. Labor is divided into three stages:

- **The first stage** occurs from the onset of true labor to full dilation of the cervix. This stage takes an average of 11 hours for a first child and 7 hours for subsequent births.

- **The second stage** occurs from the point of full dilation of the cervix to delivery of the infant. This stage takes about 1 hour for a first child and 30 to 40 minutes for subsequent births. The second stage may be longer if you have an epidural (see the "Regional anesthetics" section later in this chapter for more on epidurals).

- **The third stage** occurs from the time of delivery of the baby to delivery of the placenta — usually less than 20 minutes for all deliveries.

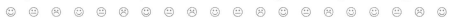
The first stage

The first stage of labor is by far the longest, and it is divided into three phases: the early (or latent) phase, the active phase, and the transition phase. Each phase has its own unique characteristics.

Early or latent phase

The entire early phase of the first stage of labor lasts an average of 6 to 7 hours in a first birth and 4 to 5 hours for subsequent births. But the length of labor is unpredictable, because knowing when labor actually begins is difficult.

During the early phase of the first stage of labor, contractions occur every 5 to 20 minutes in the beginning, and they increase in frequency until they are less than 5 minutes apart. The contractions last between 30 and 45 seconds at first, but as the first phase continues, they last up to 60 to 90 seconds in length. During the early phase, your cervix gradually dilates to 3 to 4 centimeters and becomes 100 percent effaced (thinned out).

In the beginning, your contractions may feel like menstrual cramps, with or without back pain. Your membranes may rupture, and you may have a bloody show. If you have been admitted to the hospital, your doctor may use a small plastic hook to rupture your membranes for you, in order to help things along.

 Early on in this phase, many women are most comfortable at home. Some have an overwhelming desire to clean or to perform other household chores. If you're hungry, eat a light meal (soup, juice, or toast, for example), but not a very heavy one because you may need anesthesia later to deal with labor complications. Time your contractions if you want to, but don't be obsessive about it. Many women find that walking around makes them more comfortable and distracts them from the pain during this early part of labor. Others prefer to rest in bed.

Active phase

The active phase of labor is usually shorter and more predictable than the early phase. For a first child, it lasts 5 hours on average. For subsequent babies, it lasts about 4 hours. Contractions occur every 3 to 5 minutes, and last about 45 to 60 seconds. Your cervix dilates from 4 to 8 or 9 centimeters.

You may feel increasing discomfort or pain during this phase, and you may get a backache, as well. By this time, you're probably already in the hospital or birthing center. Some patients prefer to rest in bed; others would rather walk around. Unless your practitioner asks you to stay in bed so that you can be monitored, do whatever makes you comfortable. This is the time to use the breathing and relaxation techniques you practiced in childbirth class (see Chapter 6).

Transition phase

During the transition phase, contractions occur every 2 to 3 minutes and last about 60 seconds. The contractions during this phase are very intense. Your cervix dilates from 8 or 9 to 10 centimeters. Note that many practitioners consider this transition period part of the active phase.

In addition to very intense contractions, you may notice an increase in bloody show and increased pressure, especially on your rectum, as the baby's head descends. During this last phase of the first stage of labor, you may feel as if you want to have a bowel movement. Don't worry; this sensation is a good sign and indicates that the fetus is heading in the right direction.

If you feel the urge to push, let your practitioner know. You may be fully dilated, but try not to push until you're told to do so. Pushing before you're fully dilated can slow the labor process or tear your cervix.

 Practice breathing exercises and relaxation techniques if they work for you. When you want pain medication or an epidural anesthetic (both described in the "Regional anesthetics" section later in this chapter), let your practitioner know. He or she decides which pain relief options are best for you based on how far along in labor you are and other factors related to your health and your baby's health.

Potential problems during the first stage of labor

Most women experience the first stage of labor without any problems. But if a problem arises, here is some information to help you handle it with a clear, focused mind:

⚕ **Prolonged early (latent) phase:** The early phase of labor is considered prolonged if it lasts more than 20 hours in a woman having her first child or more than 14 hours in a woman who has delivered a previous child. One approach for handling a prolonged early phase is to use medication, such as a sedative, to help you relax. The other approach is to try to move labor along by performing an *amniotomy* (rupturing the membranes or breaking your water) or by administering oxytocin (see the "Oxytocin" sidebar earlier in this chapter).

❀ **Protraction disorders:** Protraction disorders can occur if the cervix dilates too slowly or if the baby's head doesn't descend at a normal rate. These disorders may be caused by a poor fit between the baby's head and the mother's birth canal (called *cephalopelvic disproportion,* or CPD). Protraction disorders may also occur because the baby's head is in an unfavorable position or because the number or intensity of contractions is inadequate. In both cases, many practitioners administer oxytocin to improve labor progress.

❀ **Arrest disorders:** Arrest disorders occur if the cervix stops dilating or if the baby's head stops descending for more than two hours during active labor. Arrest disorders are often associated with CPD, but an infusion of oxytocin may solve the problem. If oxytocin doesn't alleviate the arrest disorder, you may need a cesarean section.

The second and third stages

The second stage of labor begins when you are fully dilated (at 10 centimeters) and ends with the delivery of your baby. This is the "pushing" stage and, although technically it is part of labor, it is described in detail in Chapter 8. The third stage begins when the baby is out and ends with the delivery of the placenta. You can find more detail about this stage in Chapter 8.

Managing the Pain of Labor

During the first stage of labor, pain is caused by contractions of the uterus and dilation of the cervix. The pain may feel like severe menstrual cramps at first, but in the second stage of labor, the stretching of the birth canal as the baby passes through it adds a different kind of pain — often a great feeling of pressure on the lower pelvis or rectum. Thanks to well-practiced breathing and relaxation exercises, along with modern techniques of anesthesia, the pain needn't be excruciating.

Most practitioners acknowledge that labor is inherently painful even for women who have diligently attended childbirth classes. The degree of pain varies from woman to woman, as does the willingness and ability to tolerate pain. Some women choose to deal with the pain on their own or with the help of breathing and distraction techniques learned in childbirth classes. Other women want medication to help them deal with the pain, no matter how well prepared they are.

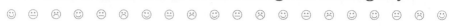
 Don't feel that you're in any way falling short of being a perfect mother or that your pregnancy is not "natural" if you need medication to help with labor pain. Everyone responds to pain differently, both emotionally and physiologically, so even if your best friend, sister, or mother got through labor with little or no pain medication, you aren't failing yourself if you choose to use it. Look at it this way: Women who are in excruciating pain usually don't breathe regularly. They also tense their muscles, and by doing so, they may prolong labor. They also tend to thrash around, making monitoring the baby difficult.

Systemic medications

The most common medications used systemically are relatives of the narcotic morphine — drugs such as meperidine (brand name Demerol), fentanyl (Sublimaze), butorphanal (Stadol), and nalbuphine (Nubain). These medications can be given every 2 to 4 hours as needed, either intravenously (through an IV) or intramuscularly (with a shot). Giving them intravenously brings pain relief more quickly, often in as little as five to ten minutes, but when the medicine is given intravenously, the pain relief doesn't last as long as it does when the medication is injected into a muscle. Also, medication given intravenously sometimes causes a greater drop in blood pressure. Intramuscular injections give longer-lasting pain relief because the medication is released into the circulating blood more slowly. But you may need to wait as long as 20 or 30 minutes before you feel any relief from pain. Many doctors use a combination of the two methods in order to provide both fast-acting and long-lasting pain relief.

 Medications you take have side effects, and pain relievers used during labor are no exception. Nausea, vomiting, drowsiness, and a drop in blood pressure are the main side effects for the mother. The degree to which the fetus or newborn is affected depends on how close to the time of delivery the medication is given.

Regional anesthetics

Systemic medications are distributed via the bloodstream to all parts of the body. Yet most of the pain of labor and delivery is concentrated in the uterus, vagina, and rectum. For that reason, regional anesthesia is sometimes used to deliver pain medication to those specific areas. Commonly used techniques for administering regional pain relief include epidural anesthesia, spinal anesthesia, caudal and saddle blocks, and pudendal blocks. These techniques are explained here.

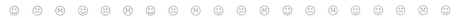

❀ **Epidural anesthesia:** Epidural anesthesia is perhaps the most popular form of pain relief for labor. Women who have had it often say, "Why didn't I get this earlier?" or "Why was I hesitant about this?" In an epidural, a tiny, flexible, plastic catheter is inserted through a needle into your lower back and threaded into the space above the membrane covering the spinal cord. For most women, this process isn't painful at all. After the catheter is in place, medication can be sent through it to numb the nerves coming from the lower part of the spine — nerves that go to the uterus, vagina, and perineum. The catheter (not the needle) stays in place throughout labor in case you need what's called a *top up* dose of the anesthetic to get you through the rest of labor and delivery. An epidural must be administered by an anesthesiologist with special training in epidural catheter placement, so epidurals may not be available in every hospital.

❀ **Spinal anesthesia:** Spinal anesthesia is similar to an epidural but different in that the medication is injected into the space *under* the membrane covering the spinal cord, rather than above it. This technique is often used for cesarean delivery, especially when a cesarean is needed suddenly, and no epidural was placed during labor.

❀ **Caudal and saddle blocks:** Caudal blocks and saddle blocks involve placing medications very low in the spinal canal. As such, they affect only those pain nerves going to the vagina and *perineum* (the area between the vagina and anus). Caudal blocks get their name because they are placed in the *caudal,* or lower, part of the spinal canal. Saddle blocks are so named because the area that is anesthetized is the same area of your legs and groin that comes in contact with a saddle when you sit in it. In both methods, pain relief comes rapidly, but the relief wears off sooner than it does with other anesthetics. Placing these blocks also requires significant expertise on the part of the anesthesiologist. They aren't available everywhere.

❀ **Pudendal blocks:** Your doctor can place a pudendal block by injecting an anesthetic inside the vagina, in the area next to the pudendal nerves. This technique numbs part of the vagina and the perineum, but it does nothing to relieve the pain from contractions.

General anesthesia

When you have general anesthesia, you are made fully unconscious by an anesthesiologist using a variety of medications. Doctors almost never use this technique for labor anymore. It is used (but only rarely) for cesarean deliveries because it is associated with a higher risk of complications. Of course, you sleep through the delivery of your baby under general anesthesia. But if, in a cesarean delivery, you have a clotting problem that rules out placing a needle into your spinal column, or if the cesarean is an emergency and there isn't enough time to place an epidural, general anesthesia should be used.

89

Chapter 8

Thirty Minutes or Less? Doubtful! The Delivery

Most expectant mothers spend a great deal of the 40 weeks of pregnancy thinking ahead to the delivery. If you're having a baby for the first time, the delivery can be pretty scary. Even if you've had a child before, worrying a bit until you see your beautiful baby is perfectly normal. When you reach the end of the second stage of labor (see Chapter 7 for details on the stages of labor), you are very, very close to the point of delivery. It's time to trust yourself, and let this natural process move along one step at a time. This chapter describes the basic process of childbirth, both vaginal and cesarean deliveries, to try to give you a clear and fairly detailed picture of what's going to happen when you're in labor.

Babies are delivered in one of three ways: through the birth canal by your pushing, through the birth canal with a little assistance (that is, using forceps or a vacuum extractor), or by cesarean delivery. The method that's right for you depends on many different factors, including your medical history, the baby's condition, and the size of your pelvis relative to the size of your baby.

Having a Vaginal Delivery

The most common method of delivery is, of course, a vaginal delivery, as shown in Figure 8-1. Most women experience what doctors call a *spontaneous vaginal delivery*, which means that the delivery occurs as a result of pushing, and it proceeds without a great deal of intervention. If you do

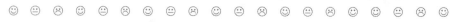
need a little help, it may come in the form of forceps or a vacuum extractor. A delivery requiring the use of one of these tools is called an *operative vaginal delivery.* This section and the next discuss both courses of events.

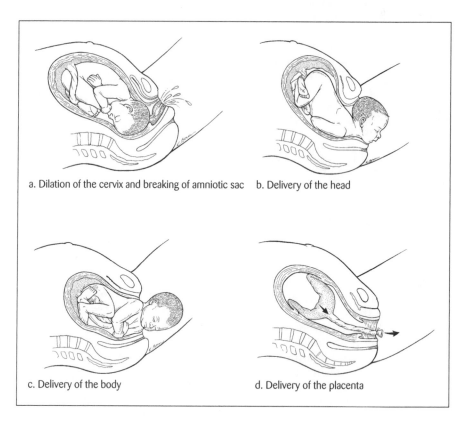

a. Dilation of the cervix and breaking of amniotic sac   b. Delivery of the head

c. Delivery of the body   d. Delivery of the placenta

Figure 8-1: An overview of the delivery process.

During the first stage of labor, your cervix dilates, and your membranes rupture. When your cervix is fully *dilated* (open to 10 centimeters), you reach the end of the first stage of labor and are ready to enter the second stage. In this stage, you push your baby through the birth canal (vagina) and actually deliver him or her.

At the end of the first stage, as the baby's head descends in the birth canal and puts pressure on neighboring internal organs, you may feel an overwhelming sensation of pressure on your rectum. You may feel as if you need to have a bowel movement. This sensation is usually strongest during contractions. If you have an epidural (see Chapter 7), you may not feel this pressure, but if you do feel it, let your nurse or practitioner know. Your cervix is getting close to being fully dilated, and it may be time for you to push. (Your nurse or doctor performs an internal exam to confirm that your cervix is fully dilated. If it is, he or she tells you to start pushing.)

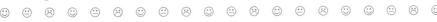

Pushing the baby out

Depending on the baby's position and size, whether you have an epidural (see Chapter 7), and whether you've had children before, pushing usually takes 30 to 90 minutes (though sometimes it takes as long as three hours). Your nurse or practitioner gives you instructions on how to push. While you're pushing, your baby moves farther along its downward course. Women often begin pushing when the baby's head is at a station of –1 or zero (mid-range). Pushing continues until the baby is at the lowest station, +3 or +5, depending on which scale your practitioner uses (see Chapter 7 for an explanation of *station*). At this stage, you can usually deliver the baby's head with one or two additional pushes.

You have several possible positions in which to push. The most common is the lithotomy position. In this position, you lean back and pull your flexed knees to your chest. At the same time, you bend your neck and try to touch your chin to your chest. The idea is to get your body to form a C. It's not the most flattering position in the world, but it does help to align the uterus and pelvis in a position that makes delivery relatively easy.

Other positions are the squatting or knee-chest variations. The advantage of squatting is that gravity works with you. A disadvantage is that you may be too tired to hold the position very long, and any monitoring equipment or an intravenous line you may have can be cumbersome. The knee-chest position is one in which you push while on all fours. This position is sometimes helpful if the baby's head is rotated in the birth canal in such a way that makes pushing the baby out in the lithotomy or squatting positions difficult. The knee-chest position may be awkward for some, however, and difficult to stay in for very long. Finding the position that feels best and works best for you may take a bit of experimentation.

When you start to feel a contraction, your nurse or doctor will likely tell you to take a deep, cleansing breath. After that, you inhale deeply again, hold in the air, and push like crazy. Focus the push toward your rectum and *perineum* (the area between the vagina and the rectum). Trying not to tense up the muscles of your vagina or rectum. Push like you're having a bowel movement. Don't worry or be embarrassed if you pass stool while you're pushing. In fact, passing stool is a sign that you're pushing correctly. Passing stool is the rule rather than the exception, and all the people helping to take care of you have seen it many times before.

Try to hold each push for about ten seconds. Many nurses count to ten or ask your coach to count to ten to help you judge the time. At the count of ten, quickly release the breath you have been holding, take in another deep breath, and push again for another ten seconds, exactly as before. You push about three times with each contraction, depending on the length of the contraction.

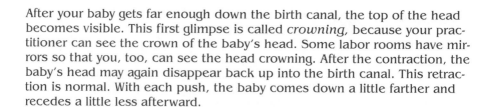

After your baby gets far enough down the birth canal, the top of the head becomes visible. This first glimpse is called *crowning*, because your practitioner can see the crown of the baby's head. Some labor rooms have mirrors so that you, too, can see the head crowning. After the contraction, the baby's head may again disappear back up into the birth canal. This retraction is normal. With each push, the baby comes down a little farther and recedes a little less afterward.

Getting an episiotomy

Just before it's born, the baby's head pushes out the *perineum* (the area between the vagina and the rectum) and stretches the skin around the vagina. As the baby's head comes through the opening of the vagina, it may tear the tissues in the back, or *posterior*, part of the vaginal opening, sometimes even to the point that the tear extends into the rectum. To minimize tearing of the surrounding skin and perineal muscles, your practitioner may make an *episiotomy* — a cut in the posterior part of the vaginal opening large enough to allow the baby's head to come through with minimal tearing or to provide extra room for delivery.

Whether you need an episiotomy can't be decided until the head is almost out. Some doctors routinely make episiotomies; others wait to see whether it's definitely necessary. Episiotomies are more common in women having their first baby than in those who have delivered before. In addition, the type of episiotomy — *median* or *mediolateral* — made may depend on your body, on the position of the baby's head, or on the judgment of your practitioner.

Prolonged second stage

If you're having your first child and you remain in the second stage of labor for more than 2 hours (or 3 hours if you have an epidural), the labor is considered prolonged. If you are having your second or subsequent child, a second stage nearing 1 hour (or 2 hours if you have an epidural) is also considered prolonged.

A prolonged second stage may be due to inadequate contractions or to *cephalopelvic disproportion*, the inability of the baby's head to pass through the mother's pelvis. Sometimes, the baby's head is in a position that blocks further descent. Oxytocin, a synthetic hormone similar to one that your body naturally releases during labor, may help to induce labor. Your practitioner may try to rotate the baby's head. You may also try changing your position to push more effectively. Sometimes forceps do the trick if the baby's head is low enough in the birth canal (see the "Having an Operative Vaginal Delivery" section later in this chapter). If all else fails, your doctor may recommend a cesarean delivery, which is discussed in the "Having a Cesarean Delivery" section later in this chapter.

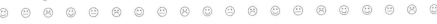

Delivery at last!

When the baby's head remains visible between contractions, your nurse helps get you into position to deliver. If you're in a birthing room, all that needs to be done is to remove the platform at the foot of your bed and set up padded leg supports. If you need to be moved to a delivery room (more like an operating room), your nurse moves you and all your monitors to a stretcher. Whether you deliver in a birthing or a delivery room depends on the facility and on any risk factors you may have.

You still have to keep pushing with each of your contractions. Your doctor or nurse cleans your perineum, usually with an iodine solution, and places drapes over your legs to keep the area as clean as possible for the new-born. As you push, your perineum gets more and more stretched out. Whether you need an episiotomy (described in the "Getting an episiotomy" section earlier in this chapter) is usually determined at the final moments. If it seems that you will otherwise tear the perineum or rectal area, your practitioner may decide to make an episiotomy.

With each push, the baby's head descends farther and farther until, finally, it comes out of the birth canal. After the baby's head delivers, your practitioner tells you to stop pushing so that he or she can suction secretions from the baby's mouth and nose.

 To stop pushing at this point can be difficult because of the intense pressure in your perineal area; panting may make it a little easier not to push. If you have an epidural, on the other hand, you may not feel this intense pressure.

Your practitioner also checks at this point to see whether the umbilical cord is wrapped around the baby's neck. A *nuchal cord,* as it's called, is actually quite common and not a cause for concern. Your practitioner simply removes the loop from around the baby's neck before delivering the rest of the baby.

After the nurse suctions out your baby's mouth and checks for a nuchal cord, your practitioner instructs you to push again to deliver the baby's body. Because the head is typically the widest part, delivery of the body is usually easier. When the whole body is out, the baby's mouth and nose are suctioned again.

Your baby's first cry

Shortly after delivery, the baby takes its first breath and begins to cry. Crying expands the baby's lungs and helps clear deeper secretions. In spite of the stereotype, most practitioners don't spank a baby after it's born, but instead use another method to stimulate crying and breathing — rubbing the baby's back vigorously, for example, or tapping the bottom of the feet. Don't be surprised if your baby doesn't cry the very second after it's born. Often, several seconds, if not minutes, pass before the baby starts making that lovely sound!

Cutting the cord

The next step is to clamp and cut the umbilical cord. Your labor coach may be offered the opportunity to cut the cord, but your partner certainly doesn't have to and shouldn't if he or she doesn't want to. If having the opportunity to cut the cord is something you feel strongly about, let your practitioner know ahead of time.

After cutting the cord, your practitioner either lays your baby on your abdomen or hands the baby to your labor nurse to put under an infant warmer. The choice depends on your baby's condition, your doctor's or nurse's standard practice, and on the policies of the facility where you're delivering.

Appearance of your baby

Often, a baby comes out covered with some blood or *vernix,* a thick, white substance that a nurse cleans off. Depending on how your labor progressed and on how long you pushed, your baby may also have a bit of a conehead, a normal response to childbirth that disappears in one to two days. It happens as the baby's head molds to fit through the birth canal. The little knit caps that most babies wear to prevent heat loss often make the shape unnoticeable.

Delivering the placenta

After the baby is born, the third stage of delivery begins — the delivery of the placenta, also known as the *afterbirth* (refer to Figure 8-1d). This stage lasts only 5 to 15 minutes. You still have contractions, but they are much less intense. These contractions help separate the placenta from the wall of the uterus. After this separation occurs and the placenta reaches the opening of the vagina, you may be asked to give one more gentle push. Many women, exhilarated by and exhausted from the delivery, pay little attention to this part of the process and later on don't even remember it.

After the placenta is out, your practitioner inspects your cervix, vagina, and perineum for tears or damage. The episiotomy or any tears are then repaired by stitching. If you didn't have an epidural and you have sensation in your perineum, your practitioner may use a local anesthetic to numb the area before repairing it. These tears are graded, according to the degree of

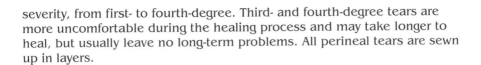
severity, from first- to fourth-degree. Third- and fourth-degree tears are more uncomfortable during the healing process and may take longer to heal, but usually leave no long-term problems. All perineal tears are sewn up in layers.

Shaking after delivery

Almost immediately after delivery, most women start to shake uncontrollably. You need not be concerned at all about this shaking. It usually goes away within a few hours after delivery. Your partner may think that you are cold and offer you a blanket. Blankets do help some women, but you really are not shivering because you're cold. The cause of this phenomenon is unclear, but it is nearly universal — even among women who have cesarean deliveries.

 Some women feel nervous about holding their babies because they are shaking so much. If you feel this way, let your partner or your nurse hold your baby until you feel up to it.

Having an Operative Vaginal Delivery

If the baby's head is low enough in the birth canal and your practitioner feels that the baby needs to be delivered immediately or that you won't be able to deliver the baby vaginally without some added help, he or she may recommend the use of forceps or a vacuum extractor to assist the delivery. A delivery with either of these instruments is called an *operative vaginal delivery*. It may be appropriate to use when

* You've pushed for a long time, and you're too tired to continue pushing hard enough to deliver.

* You've pushed for some time, and your practitioner thinks you won't deliver vaginally unless you have this type of help.

* The baby's heart rate pattern indicates a need to deliver the baby quickly.

* The baby's position is making it very difficult for you to push it out on your own.

As shown in Figure 8-2, *forceps* are two curved, spatula-like instruments that are placed on the sides of the baby's head to help guide it through the outer part of the birth canal. The *vacuum extractor* is a suction cup placed on the top of the baby's head. Suction is applied to allow your practitioner to gently pull the baby through the birth canal.

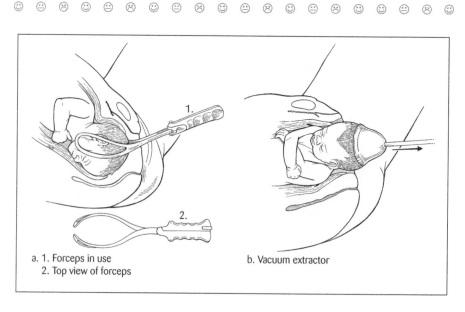

a. 1. Forceps in use
   2. Top view of forceps

b. Vacuum extractor

Figure 8-2: Two ways to help a vaginal delivery.

Either technique is safe for both you and the baby if the baby is far enough down the birth canal and the instruments are used appropriately. In fact, these techniques can often help avoid a cesarean delivery. The decision to use forceps or a vacuum often depends upon the judgment and experience of your practitioner and the position and station of the baby.

Having a Cesarean Delivery

Many patients wonder whether they'll need a cesarean. Sometimes your doctor knows the answer before labor even begins because you have *placenta previa* (where the placenta partially or wholly covers the cervix), for example, or the baby is in a *transverse lie* (the baby is lying sideways within the uterus rather than head-down). But most of the time, the decision to have a cesarean can't be made until you see how your labor progresses and how your baby tolerates labor. A cesarean delivery that is planned ahead is called an *elective* cesarean.

Because a cesarean is a surgical procedure, it's always performed by a doctor. All nurse-midwives and many family-practice doctors work with an obstetrician in case their patients need a cesarean. Some family-practice physicians have also had the special training needed to perform cesarean deliveries.

If your practitioner feels that you need a cesarean delivery, he or she will discuss it with you. In cases in which the baby is in a *breech position,* with the head facing up instead of down, you and your practitioner may consider together the pros and cons of having either an elective cesarean delivery or a vaginal breech delivery. Both carry some risks, and often your practitioner asks which risks are most acceptable to you. If the decision to perform a cesarean is due to a last-minute emergency, the discussion between you and your doctor may happen quickly, while you're being wheeled to the operating room.

A cesarean delivery is performed in an operating room under sterile conditions. An intravenous line must be in place and a catheter put in the bladder. After your abdomen is scrubbed with antiseptic solution, sterile sheets are placed over your belly. One of the sheets is elevated to create a screen so that the expectant parents don't have to watch the procedure.

The exact place on the woman's abdomen where the incision is made depends on the reason she's having the cesarean. Usually, it is low, just above the pubic bone, in a transverse direction (perpendicular to the torso). This cut is known as a *Pfannensteil incision* or, more commonly, a bikini cut. Less often, the incision is vertical, along the midline of the abdomen.

All surgical procedures involve risks, and cesarean delivery is no exception. Fortunately, these problems are not common. The main risks of cesarean delivery are

❀ Excessive bleeding, rarely to the point of needing a blood transfusion

❀ Development of an infection in the uterus, bladder, or skin incision

❀ Injury to the bladder, bowel, or adjacent organs

❀ Development of blood clots in the legs or pelvis after the operation

Other than the fact that the baby and placenta are delivered through an incision in the uterus rather than the vagina, how the baby is delivered doesn't matter to the baby. Babies delivered by a cesarean before labor usually don't have the coneheads discussed in the "Appearance of your baby" section earlier in this chapter. Yours may have a conehead, however if you're in labor for a long time before having the cesarean.

Anesthesia for a cesarean delivery

The most common forms of anesthesia used for cesarean deliveries are epidural and spinal (see Chapter 7 for more information about anesthesia). Both kinds of anesthesia numb you from mid-chest to toes but also allow you to remain awake so that you can experience the birth of your child. You may feel some tugging and pulling during the operation, but you do not feel pain. Sometimes, the anesthesiologist injects a slow-release pain

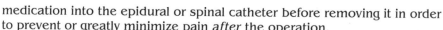
medication into the epidural or spinal catheter before removing it in order to prevent or greatly minimize pain *after* the operation.

If the baby has to be delivered in an emergency and there's no time to place an epidural or spinal, general anesthesia may be needed. In that case, you are asleep during the cesarean and totally unaware of the procedure. General anesthesia may be needed in some cases due to complications in pregnancy that make it unwise to place epidurals or spinals.

Reasons for a cesarean delivery

The reasons doctors perform cesarean deliveries are many, but all have to do with delivering the infant in the safest, healthiest way possible while maintaining the mother's well-being. The following lists describe the most common reasons for cesarean deliveries.

Reasons for an elective cesarean delivery:

- Abnormal position of the baby (breech or sideways)

- *Placenta previa,* where the placenta partially or wholly covers the cervix

- Extensive prior surgery on the mother's uterus, including previous cesarean deliveries or removal of uterine fibroids

- Delivery of triplets or more

Reasons for an unplanned but non-emergency cesarean delivery include:

- The baby is too large in relation to the woman's pelvis to be delivered safely through the vagina — a condition known as *cephalopelvic disproportion* (CPD) — or the position of the baby's head makes vaginal delivery unlikely.

- Signs indicate that the baby is not tolerating labor.

- Maternal medical conditions preclude safe vaginal delivery, such as severe cardiac disease.

- Normal labor comes to a standstill.

Reasons for emergency cesarean delivery include the following:

- Bleeding is excessive.

- The baby's umbilical cord pushes through the cervix when the membranes rupture.

- The baby's heart rate has slowed down for a prolonged period of time.

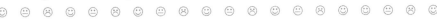

Why they call it cesarean

Cesarean delivery, in which the baby is born through an incision in the mother's abdomen, is hardly a new medical innovation. Cases have been documented since the beginning of recorded history. In fact, many famous works of medieval and Renaissance art depict abdominal deliveries.

The origin of the term *cesarean section* is a subject of some controversy. Julius Caesar, it turns out, was probably not delivered this way, according to *Cesarean Delivery,* a history written by physicians Steve Clark and Jeffrey Phelan. In those days, it was rare for the mother to survive the procedure. Yet Caesar's mother survived her delivery and was depicted in Renaissance art recounting the life of Caesar as an adult, which means that her delivery was likely vaginal.

One theory is that the name comes from the *Lex Cesare,* the laws of the ancient Roman emperors. One of those laws mandated that any woman who died while she was pregnant be delivered by an abdominal incision so that the infant could be baptized. This rule later became canon law of the Catholic church. A third possible explanation for the term *cesarean* is its relationship to the Latin term *cadere,* which means *to cut.* The term *section* also implies surgical cutting, so if *cadere* is indeed the origin of *cesarean,* then *cesarean section* is redundant. In modern obstetrics, the preferred phrase is *cesarean delivery* or *cesarean birth.* Still, many people continue to call the operation a cesarean section or *C-section.*

Recovery from a cesarean delivery

After the surgery is finished, you're taken to a recovery area, where you stay for a few hours until the hospital staff can make sure that your condition is stable. Often, you can see and hold your baby during this time.

During the first day after a cesarean, you need to spend most of the time in bed. After that, you need to gradually increase your activity, so that you can build the strength you need to take care of yourself and the baby at home. The recovery time from a cesarean delivery is usually longer than from a vaginal delivery, because the procedure is a surgical one. Typically, you stay in the hospital for two to four days — sometimes longer, if complications arise.

You may feel pain where the incisions were made through your skin and uterus. Ask your nurse for pain medication if you need it. Your doctor usually leaves orders for pain medications, but they aren't automatically given unless you ask for them. The anesthesia needed to perform a cesarean delivery also tends to slow the bowels and to cause some bloating and abdominal discomfort. Again, medications can help, as can prune juice and other juices. *Lochia* (bleeding) may also come from the vagina, just like in a vaginal delivery. This discharge gradually decreases and eventually disappears.

Women who have labored for a long time only to find that they need a cesarean delivery are sometimes, understandably, disappointed. This reaction is natural. If it happens to you, keep in mind that your safety and the safety of your baby are what really matter. Having a cesarean delivery doesn't mean that you are a failure or that you didn't try hard enough. Practitioners stick to established guidelines when monitoring progress through labor, and those guidelines are all about giving you and your baby the best chance for a normal, healthy outcome.

Congratulations! You Did It!

After her baby is born, a woman may experience any and every kind of emotion. The spectrum of feelings is truly infinite. Most of the time, you're completely overcome with joy when your long-awaited baby finally is born. You may be incredibly relieved to see that your baby appears healthy and okay. If your baby requires extra medical attention for some reason and you can't hold him or her right away, you may be upset or, at the very least, disappointed. Just remember that very soon, you'll have him or her to hold and enjoy for the rest of your life. Some women feel too scared or overwhelmed to care for their babies right away. Don't feel guilty about such feelings — they, and most other feelings, are completely normal. Just take it one moment at a time. You've come through a phenomenal event.

Causes for Concern

Childbirth may not be the easiest thing a woman ever does in her life, but in the vast majority of cases, it occurs in a fairly predictable way that causes no problems for the mother or the baby. However, in some cases, the delivery gets complicated. Here are three problems that occur in a minority of pregnancies:

✸ **Lacerations to the birth canal:** Most tears or lacerations that occur during delivery are in the perineum (the area between the vagina and rectum) or are extensions of an episiotomy, which is also in that area. Especially if the baby is exceptionally large or you have an operative vaginal delivery, lacerations occasionally occur in other areas, such as the cervix, the walls of the vagina, the labia, or the tissue around the urethra. Your practitioner examines the birth canal carefully after delivery and sews up any lacerations that need to be repaired. These lacerations usually heal quickly and almost never cause long-term problems.

Chapter 8: Thirty Minutes or Less? Doubtful! The Delivery

☺ ☺ ☹ ☺ ☺ ☹ ☺ ☺ ☹ ☺ ☺ ☹ ☺ ☺ ☹ ☺ ☺ ☺ ☹ ☺

❀ **Postpartum bleeding:** After delivery, the uterus begins to contract in order to squeeze the blood vessels closed and thus slow down bleeding. If the uterus doesn't contract normally, excessive bleeding may occur. This condition is known as *uterine atony.* Your doctor or nurse may first massage your uterus to get it to contract. If massage doesn't solve the problem, you may be given one of several medications — oxytocin, methergine, or Hemabate — that promotes contracting. If some placental material remains in your uterus, it may need to be removed by reaching inside the uterus or by a *D&C* (dilation and curettage), which involves scraping the lining of the uterus with an instrument.

❀ **Shoulder dystocia:** After the baby's head delivers, the shoulders and body follow easily. Occasionally, though, the baby's shoulders get stuck behind the mother's pubic bone, which makes delivery of the rest of the baby more difficult. This situation is known as *shoulder dystocia.* If you have this problem, your practitioner can perform various maneuvers to dislodge the shoulders and deliver the baby.

Chapter 9

The First Few Days with Your Brand-New Baby

For 40 weeks, you and your baby have been in one body. If you're like most women, you've focused on staying healthy to help your baby grow and on preparing to deliver your baby safely. But suddenly, your baby is out on his own, and you finally get to take your first real look at him. Newborns typically look a little funny and may even have a cone-shaped head, blotches, and a white, pasty goo — all traits that will soon disappear.

This chapter lets you know what you can expect your baby to look like and also how he or she is cared for in the hospital. Medical tests are conducted (usually nothing too strenuous), your baby is cleaned up, and you make your first efforts at breast-feeding, if you so choose. This chapter also covers various minor health problems your baby may experience and lets you know how the hospital's medical staff deals with them. Finally, you get tried-and-true tips for managing those first days with your new baby at home.

Love at First Sight

Immediately after delivery, your practitioner either puts your baby on your belly or hands your baby to your nurse for some judicious cleansing and toweling off before putting the baby in your arms.

In the first moments after your baby is born, you may be overwhelmed by feelings of love. You may also be dazed by the shock and relief of it all. Most likely, you will think that your baby is the most beautiful thing you've ever seen. But contrary to the fairy tales you see on TV soap operas, *I Love Lucy* reruns, and cartoons, babies don't always come out clean and smelling like a spring shower. Newborns are often covered with some of your blood, amniotic fluid, and a white goo known as *vernix*. The baby's skin may be blotchy. He or she may even have suffered a few bruises during delivery. So keep an open mind when assessing his or her appearance right off the bat.

Some women feel a little hesitant at first or overwhelmed at the sight of their newborn baby. Often it takes a few days to establish a true connection or bond with your baby. If you are feeling like this, don't worry. As reality sets in and you get to know your baby, you'll feel much better.

Vernix caseosa

A thick, white, waxy substance typically covers a newborn baby from head to toe. The formal name for this substance is *vernix caseosa,* a phrase whose Latin roots mean "cheesy varnish." Vernix is a mixture of cells that have sloughed off from the outer layer of the baby's skin and debris from the amniotic fluid. Some doctors believe that vernix acts as an emollient to protect the tender fetal skin from the dryness that may result from living within a bag of amniotic fluid. Others believe that the vernix acts as a lubricant to help the baby slide through the birth canal. Some babies have more vernix than others; some have none at all. Whatever vernix doesn't come off when the nurses dry your baby is usually absorbed within the first 24 hours.

Caput and molding

Caput succedaneum — more commonly called *caput* — refers to a circular area of swelling on the baby's head, located at the spot that pushed against the opening to the cervix during delivery. The swollen area ranges in size from only a few millimeters in diameter to several centimeters (a few inches). Caput generally disappears within 24 to 48 hours after birth.

Babies who are born head-first *(vertex)* often go through a process known as *molding.* Molding occurs because, throughout labor, as the baby descends through the birth canal, it "fits" its way along. Molding doesn't cause any harm. The bones and soft tissues in the baby's head are designed to allow molding to happen. The result is often a baby with a cone-shaped head. By 24 hours after delivery, the molding is usually gone, and the baby's head appears round and smooth. Babies born in the breech presentation, babies born by cesarean, and babies born to a woman who has had children before may not have molding.

During the passage through the birth canal, a baby's ears can fold down into strange positions. The same thing can happen with the baby's nose, so that, at first, it may appear *asymmetric,* or pushed to one side. But these features are no reason to rush your baby to a plastic surgeon. These minor oddities are temporary and disappear in a few days.

Black and blue marks

Quite often, babies are born with black-and-blue marks on their heads from the labor and delivery process. These marks appear because the forces of labor put so much pressure on the baby's scalp, or as a result of a forceps or vacuum delivery. A bruise doesn't indicate that anything harmful has occurred. Most black-and-blue marks go away within the first few days of life.

Blotches, patches, and other skin-deep characteristics

Most people think of newborn skin as blemish-free, the very definition of perfection. But at first, babies have all kinds of spots and markings — most of which disappear within a matter of days or weeks. Here are some of the most common skin conditions that affect newborns:

* **Neonatal acne:** Some babies are born with tiny white or red pimples around the nose, lips, and cheeks; some develop these pimples weeks or months later. These bumps are completely normal and are sometimes called *neonatal acne* or, in some cases, *milia.* No need to rush to the dermatologist, though. The little bumps disappear in time.

* **Stork bites:** You may notice small ruptured blood vessels on the back of the neck and around your baby's nose and eyes. These marks are commonly known as *stork bites* and *angel kisses.* They also disappear after a while, sometimes in a few weeks or months.

* **Red spots:** Reddish discoloration on the skin, whether very deep and dark or light and hardly noticeable, is common in newborns. Most of these discolorations go away or fade, but some persist as birthmarks. One type in particular, *erythema taxicum,* can be extensive. It looks like bad hives, and it comes and goes over the baby's first few days of life.

* **Hemangiomas:** Another type of reddish spot, known as a *hemangioma,* may not appear until a week or so after delivery. These spots can be almost any size, large or small, and can occur anywhere on the infant's body. The majority go away in early childhood, but some persist. Hemangiomas that become bothersome (because of their appearance) can be treated. You can discuss treatment options with your pediatrician.

❀ **Mongolian spots:** Bluish-gray patches of skin on the lower back, buttocks, and thighs are especially common in Asian, Southern European, and African-American infants. These patches are sometimes called *mongolian spots.* They usually disappear in early childhood.

❀ **Dry skin:** Some babies, particularly those who are born late, have an outer layer of skin that looks shriveled like a raisin and peels off easily shortly after birth. You can use lotion or oil, if needed, as a moisturizer.

Baby hair

Some babies enter the world totally bald; others look as though they need a haircut. Typically, newborn hair thins out and is replaced by new hair, sometimes of a different color. Babies grow hair at different rates. Some have relatively little hair even at a year of age, while others already need a trip to the beauty salon.

Some babies are born covered by a soft, fine layer of dark hair that can be especially prominent on the forehead, shoulders, and back. This hair is called *lanugo.* It is quite normal. Lanugo is most common in preterm babies and in infants of mothers who have diabetes. It falls out in several weeks.

Newborn extremities

Newborn babies often assume a position similar to the one that they had inside the uterus, the so-called *fetal position.* You may notice that your baby likes to curl up with his or her arms and legs bent and fingers balled into a fist.

Watch out for those nails, though! Newborn fingernails and toenails can be surprisingly long and sharp. To keep newborns from scratching themselves, many hospitals dress them in little shirts with mitten-like attachments that cover the hands. It is important to keep babies' nails relatively short. Pick up a pair of baby nail scissors or clippers from your local drug store.

 A good time to trim fingernails and toenails is when your baby is fast asleep and oblivious to what you're doing.

Newborn eyes and ears

At birth, a baby's vision is quite limited. Newborns can only see objects at a distance of about 7 to 8 inches. They also respond to light and appear to be interested in bright objects.

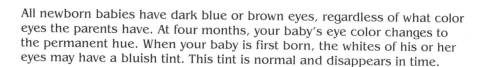

All newborn babies have dark blue or brown eyes, regardless of what color eyes the parents have. At four months, your baby's eye color changes to the permanent hue. When your baby is first born, the whites of his or her eyes may have a bluish tint. This tint is normal and disappears in time.

Some newborns' eyes appear a little swollen or puffy. This puffiness is caused by the delivery process; it is perfectly normal, and it quickly subsides. Some puffiness may also be due to antibiotic put in the eyes after birth (see the "Eye care" section later in this chapter).

Babies are fully able to hear from the moment they are born, which is why you may notice that your baby reacts with a startled motion to loud or sudden noises. Newborns also can distinguish various tastes and smells.

Newborn external genitalia and breasts

Babies are often born with a swollen or puffy scrotum or labia. The breasts may appear slightly enlarged. This swelling is caused by maternal hormones that cross the placenta. Sometimes, high maternal hormone levels even cause the baby to secrete whitish or pinkish discharge from the breasts (known as *witch's milk*) or, in females, from the vagina. These secretions are normal and transient; they go away within a few weeks after birth.

Umbilical cord

The stump of your baby's umbilical cord probably has a little piece of plastic attached to it. After delivery, the cord is closed with a small plastic clamp and then cut. Usually, this clamp is removed before you take the baby home. Then the umbilical cord stump quickly dries up and shrivels so that it looks like a hard, dark cord. Within one to three weeks, the stump usually falls off on its own. Don't try to pull it off yourself.

 To keep the stump clean, dip a cotton swab in water, alcohol, or peroxide and clean around the base. However, some pediatricians think this cleaning is unnecessary unless a lot of goopy stuff is around the base.

Newborn size

In general, newborn babies weigh between 6 and 8 pounds (about 2,700 to 3,600 grams) and measure between 18 to 22 inches (46 to 56 centimeters). The exact size depends on the baby's gestational age (basically, the number of weeks the pregnancy lasted), genetics, and factors such as whether the mother had diabetes, whether she smoked, and how healthy her diet was during pregnancy.

You may notice that your baby's head seems disproportionately large compared to his or her body. This is true of all newborns. It takes time for the baby to develop muscles strong enough to support the head and hold it up without assistance. You also may notice soft spots on the back and top of your baby's head. These are *fontanelles,* areas where the baby's skull bones meet. Fontanelles serve an important purpose — they allow for the rapid growth of the baby's brain. The back spot *(posterior fontanelle)* usually closes within a few months, but the *anterior or top fontanelle* (the one most typically called the *soft spot)* usually remains until the baby is 10 months to 1 year old.

Baby's first cry

Often, the baby starts to cry spontaneously shortly after delivery, but not every baby cries right away. A full-throated cry is music to the ears of everyone on the hospital staff because it triggers the baby's first breathing efforts. Healthy breathing can begin without a loud cry, however, and some babies give only a little whimper. Some have normal respiration even if they don't wail at high decibels. If your baby passed *meconium* — fecal matter from the baby that is discharged at birth — during labor, your practitioner suctions out the baby's lungs before he or she even has a chance to cry, in order to prevent the baby from breathing meconium into the lungs. Contrary to the movie stereotype, your practitioner is unlikely to turn your baby upside down and give him or her a little spank on the behind to elicit that first cry. If your baby is slow to start breathing, the doctor, nurse, or midwife will stimulate your baby by rubbing her back, by drying him off, or by tapping her feet.

Most babies breathe 30 to 40 times a minute. A newborn's respiratory rate also can increase with physical activity. Newborns breathe through their noses rather than their mouths. This great natural adaptation enables them to breathe while nursing or bottle-feeding.

Baby's First Test

All babies are evaluated by the *Apgar score,* named for Dr. Virginia Apgar, who devised it in 1952. This score is a useful way of quickly assessing the baby's initial condition to see whether he or she needs special medical attention. Five factors are measured: heart rate, respiratory effort, muscle tone, presence of reflexes, and color. Each factor is given a score of 0, 1, or 2, with 2 being the highest score. Apgar scores are calculated at one and five minutes. An Apgar score of 6 or above is perfectly fine.

Many new parents anxiously await the results of their child's Apgar score. In fact, an Apgar score taken one minute after the baby is born indicates whether the baby needs some resuscitative measures, but is not useful in predicting long-term health. An Apgar score taken five minutes later can indicate whether resuscitative measures have been effective. Occasionally, a very low five-minute Apgar score reflects decreased oxygenation to the baby, but it correlates poorly with future health. The purpose of the Apgar score is merely to help your doctor or pediatrician identify babies who need a little extra attention.

Newborn Care in the Hospital

After your nurse and practitioner are assured that your baby is fine, the hospital staff starts cleaning up the baby and helping him or her make a comfortable transition to life outside the womb. Like butterflies emerging from their cocoons, newborns must adjust to a new state of being in various ways. Suddenly, and for the first time, they are able to breathe on their own and to see the wide world around them.

Keeping the baby warm and dry

Because body temperature drops rapidly after birth, your new baby must be kept warm and dry. If newborns become cold, their oxygen requirements increase. For this reason, a nurse dries the baby off, places him or her in a warmer or warmed bassinet, and then watches the baby's temperature closely. Often, the nurse wraps or swaddles the baby in a blanket and puts a little hat on him or her to reduce the loss of heat from the head, the site of most heat loss. When the baby gets to the nursery, he or she is usually dressed in a little shirt and then wrapped up again in a blanket.

Eye care

The staff at most hospitals routinely place an antibiotic ointment into a newborn's eyes to lower the chance that the baby will develop an infection from passage through the vagina of a mother who has chlamydia or gonorrhea. The ointment doesn't appear to be bothersome to babies and is completely absorbed within a few hours.

Vitamin K

Most hospitals routinely give newborns an injection of vitamin K to decrease the risk of serious bleeding. Vitamin K is important in the body's production of *clotting factors* — substances that help the blood clot. This nutrient doesn't pass through the placenta to a baby very easily, however, and newborn livers, because they are immature, produce very little of it. So babies are typically low in this nutrient. Giving the baby vitamin K is an important preventive measure.

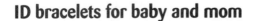
ID bracelets for baby and mom

At the hospital, your baby gets an identification bracelet to identify him or her as yours. All hospitals require the mother to wear a bracelet with the baby's ID number on it. Each time the baby is brought to the mother, the numbers are read off to ensure that the right baby is given to the right mother. Most hospitals also take additional security measures to prevent mix-ups and to prevent unauthorized individuals from gaining access to the nursery. Many nurseries are locked, and all are closely supervised.

Footprints

Most likely, footprints are taken shortly after your baby is born to make a permanent record of his or her identity. (The unique ridges that form on a baby's feet are actually present several months before birth.) Some hospitals give you a copy of your baby's footprints for your scrapbook. Although most hospitals still use this technique of identification, not all do.

Hepatitis B vaccine

Many hospitals routinely start the vaccination process against hepatitis B for newborn babies; others prefer a pediatrician to administer the first of the three shots after the baby is discharged from the hospital. (The last two are given over the course of the next six months.) Wherever it is given, this shot is an important tool to reduce the baby's chance of contracting hepatitis B later in life.

Baby's first doctor visit

Before or after delivery, someone from the hospital asks you the name of the pediatrician you have chosen to care for your baby. This doctor should be someone who is authorized to work at the hospital where you have delivered, but the doctor doesn't have to be the same pediatrician that you plan to use after you leave the hospital. If you live some distance from the hospital and have selected a pediatrician close to home who doesn't have privileges at the hospital where you deliver, you still need another pediatrician to care for your baby during the hospital stay. Depending on the time you deliver, the pediatrician may see the baby on the same day or the day after birth.

When the pediatrician examines your baby, he or she checks the baby's general appearance, listens for heart murmurs, feels the *fontanelles* (the openings in the baby's skull where the various bones come together), looks at the extremities, checks the hips, and, in general, makes sure that the baby is in good condition. The pediatrician orders a variety of standard blood tests and newborn screening tests. The screening tests required vary from state to state, but they often include tests for thyroid disease, PKU (a condition in which a person has trouble metabolizing some amino acids), and other inherited metabolic disorders. The results of these screening tests usually don't come back until after you take your baby home, so the pediatrician gives you the results at your baby's first office visit. If any of the tests come back positive, the state also notifies you by mail. Be sure to ask the pediatrician upon discharge when your baby should be seen again.

Newborn heart rate and circulatory changes

Remember how your practitioner checked the fetal heart rate during prenatal visits (see Chapters 4 through 6)? You may have noticed then how fast the beat was. In utero, the baby's heart rate is, on average, 120 to 160 beats per minute, and this heart rate pattern continues during the newborn period. Your baby's heart rate also can increase with physical activity and slow down when he or she sleeps.

After a baby is born, important changes in circulation occur. In utero, because a fetus doesn't use its lungs to breathe, much of the blood is shunted away from the lungs through a structure called the *ductus arteriosus.* Normally, this shunt closes on the first day of life. Sometimes, a murmur is heard in the first days after the baby is born, which indicates changes in blood flow. This murmur, called a PDA *(patent ductus arteriosus),* may be perfectly normal and nothing to worry about. However, some heart murmurs require further investigation in the form of a special sonogram of the baby's heart, called an *echocardiogram.* Even when murmurs due to small structural problems are found (like a small hole in the septum of the heart), many go away on their own. If your baby is diagnosed with a murmur, you should discuss it with the baby's pediatrician or a pediatric cardiologist who specializes in these conditions.

Newborn weight changes

Most newborns lose about 10 percent of their body weight during their first few days of life. Of course, if you weigh only 7 or 8 pounds (3,200 or 3,600 grams), 10 percent doesn't amount to more than a pound (454 grams). Weight loss is completely normal and is usually caused by fluid loss from urine, feces, and sweat. During the first few days of life, the typical infant takes in very little food or water to replace this weight loss. Preterm babies lose relatively more weight than full-term babies, and they may take longer to regain their weight. In contrast, babies who are small for their gestational age may gain weight more rapidly. Generally, most newborns regain their birth weight by the tenth day of life. By the age of 5 months, they're likely to double their birth weight. By the end of the first year, they triple it.

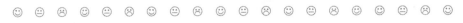
Urinating and bowel movements

The passage of bowel movements and urine is an important sign that your baby's gastrointestinal and urinary tracts are functioning well. Most babies wet their diapers six to ten times a day by the time they're 1 week old. The frequency of bowel movements depends on whether you are bottle- or breast-feeding. Typically, a breast-fed baby has two or more bowel movements per day, whereas a formula-fed baby has only one or two.

Don't be surprised if your baby's first stool looks like thick, sticky, black tar — that's normal. Ninety percent of newborns pass their first stool within the first 24 hours, and almost all the rest do so by 36 hours. Later on, the color of the stools lightens, and the texture becomes more normal. A formula-fed baby typically has semi-formed, yellow-green stools, whereas a breast-fed baby has looser, more granular, and more yellowish stools.

Newborn jaundice

When your baby is 2 to 5 days old, his or her skin may take on a yellow-orange tint. This condition is known as *physiological jaundice of the newborn,* and it develops in about one-third of all babies. Jaundice is caused by an increase in the concentration of bilirubin in the baby's blood. *Bilirubin* consists of byproducts of hemoglobin from the baby's red blood cells, byproducts that are normally disposed of through the liver and kidneys. Elevated bilirubin levels may occur because a baby's liver is not yet fully mature. Feeding the newborn early in his or her life may help to decrease the risk of jaundice, because feeding causes the baby to stay well hydrated and stimulates the digestive tract.

If jaundice occurs very early or lasts longer than usual, the pediatrician may want to check your baby's bilirubin levels daily. If bilirubin levels are high enough, the pediatrician may want to start therapy, which involves placing the baby under special phototherapy lights. This lighting helps to break up the bilirubin and causes the baby to excrete it more quickly. Keeping the baby's skin exposed to sunlight — through a window, for example — may also help to break down the bilirubin.

Bringing baby home

Finally, the day comes when you are discharged from the hospital and are able to bring your baby home. You need to bring a change of clothes for your baby to wear home. Of course, the best choice of clothes depends on whether it's summer or winter, fall or spring, or you live in a warm or cold climate. Remember that babies need frequent diaper changes, so choose clothes that are easy to open, close, put on, and take off.

Most important of all is having an infant car seat to carry your baby home in. They are eminently useful in preventing injuries to babies. In many states, you are required by law to have an infant car seat before the baby can be discharged.

In some cases, the mother is ready to leave the hospital before her baby. This can happen, for example, when a baby is born prematurely and needs time to grow and mature before leaving the hospital. It can also happen when a baby has jaundice and needs phototherapy in the hospital. Whatever the reason, going home without the new baby can cause parents to feel incredibly disappointed and empty. If this happens to you, remember that your feelings are completely normal. It's hard to go home alone after all the time you spent anticipating bringing the baby with you. Your baby will be home soon, and then you'll forget all about the first few days of separation. Your baby will be with you for a lifetime, and that includes plenty of time to build a beautiful, loving relationship. What's most important is that your baby comes home healthy!

Newborn Care at Home

On one hand, bringing your baby home is a great privilege. On the other, it is a tremendous responsibility. Suddenly, you and your partner are in charge of his or her care, without the benefit of the hospital nursing staff. Even if you have family members or a baby nurse to help, ultimately the responsibility is now yours! This section covers many of the ways in which you take care of your newborn — everything except feeding, which is discussed in Chapter 10.

Table 9-1 is a check list of items you need for your baby. Check off these items as you acquire them.

Table 9-1 A Shopping List for a Baby

✓	Items
	Baby Items
	Antibiotic cream
	Baby hairbrush
	Baby nail clippers or scissors
	Baby shampoo
	Baby soap
	Baby towels and washcloths

continued

☺ ☺ ☹ ☺ ☺ ☹ ☺ ☺ ☹ ☺ ☺ ☹ ☺ ☹ ☺ ☹ ☺ ☺ ☺ ☹ ☺

Table 9-1 A Shopping List for a Baby (continued)

✓	Items
	Bandages
	Bassinet
	Bottles for water, juice, or formula
	Changing table
	Cloth diapers (useful as burping cloths, to protect your clothes when you're bathing your baby, and to provide a clean surface on which to lay your baby)
	Crib
	Crib and bassinet sheets
	Crib bumpers (pads to put around the edges of the crib so that your baby doesn't bump his or her head on the bars)
	Detergent and fabric softener (get the kind without perfumes or dyes)
	Infant car seat
	Infant medications (anti-fever and pain-relief)
	Medicated cream for diaper rash
	Nasal aspirator (a bulb syringe for suctioning stuffy, congested noses)
	Pacifiers (some pediatricians don't advocate the use of pacifiers because of potential future orthodontic problems)
	Petroleum ointment, or some other ointment suitable for babies
	Receiving blankets
	Rectal thermometer
	Rubber pads (get two or three that you can place under the crib sheet and on the bassinet and changing table)
	Stroller (get one that adjusts to let your baby lie down)

Bathing

Until your baby's umbilical cord falls off, keep your baby clean with sponge baths only. Prepare a small container of warm water and lay your baby on the changing table or on a table or countertop padded with a towel or on one of those large sponges sold in some baby stores. With a clean wash-cloth, gently wash the baby from head to toe. Use a separate wet cotton ball for each eye. Make sure to dry your baby off right away so that he or she doesn't get cold. Because a great deal of heat is lost from the head, some mothers find it helpful to wash the head first, dry it right away, and then wash the rest of the body.

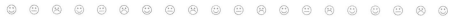

Bath tips

Bathing a squirming baby can be a little difficult, so here are some tips to help you both enjoy bath time:

* Using your elbow, test the water temperature to make sure that it isn't too hot. (Your hand may not be as sensitive to heat as your elbow is.)

* Before you put your baby in the bath, make sure that you have all your supplies: washcloth, cotton balls, mild soap if you like (washing with no soap is fine, too), mild shampoo, a dry towel, a clean diaper, and clean clothes.

* Be sure that your baby's head and body are securely supported during the bath. Remember, it will be a while before your baby can hold up his or her own head.

* Use plain water — no soap — to clean your baby's face.

* Use a washcloth to clean the outside part of the ears. Using a cotton swab inside your baby's ears or nose is not recommended.

* Wash a baby girl's genitals from front to back (to avoid washing any stool forward). For boys, clean underneath the scrotum and wash the foreskin without pulling back strongly on it.

* If your baby has very dry skin or even eczema (a condition in which the skin is chronically dry and flaky), consider bathing your baby less frequently — every other day, perhaps — because too much water can promote dryness. If it doesn't improve, talk it over with your pediatrician.

* If your baby has trouble settling down to sleep at night, you may want to consider a bath before bedtime. Your baby may find it relaxing.

* If you have twins, try bathing one baby when the other one is sleeping, so that you don't get into a situation in which you have to attend to one crying baby while you're bathing the other one.

After your baby's umbilical cord stump falls off, you're free to give him or her a bath in a tub. Many baby stores sell small plastic tubs that are designed for newborns. Some parents find it convenient to place the tub in the kitchen sink or on the counter. See the "Bath tips" sidebar in this chapter for some hints on keeping your baby clean.

 Hand-to-body contact is an easy way to transmit infections from one person to another, so make sure that people who come in contact with your baby have washed their hands well. Make sure that they wash with soap, not just water, so that their hands are as clean as possible.

Burping

Often, babies swallow air when they're feeding, especially if they're bottle-feeding. The accumulation of air inside a baby's stomach may make him or her feel uncomfortable. The good news is that all the discomfort goes away with one big burp.

 Keep a cloth diaper or burp cloth over your shoulder while burping your baby. Babies often spit up some formula or milk when burping, and the cloth protects your clothes.

Sleeping

Here are a few pointers on dealing with your baby's sleeping habits:

- Pediatricians recommend that babies sleep on their backs — not on their stomachs — because sleeping on the stomach (called the *prone position*) has been associated with sudden infant death syndrome (SIDS). To keep your baby turned on his or her back, you can roll up a blanket and use it as a prop or wedge that prevents the baby from rolling over. Infant stores sell special small cushions designed for this purpose, too.

- You may want to keep bright pictures or hanging objects around the crib to give your baby something interesting to look at when he or she is lying awake. But be careful not to place pillows or stuffed toys inside the crib or bassinet, in order to minimize any risk of suffocation.

- Playing soft music before a nap may help your baby get into the mood for sleep.

- Some babies fall asleep more easily when they're rocked to sleep. Be aware, however, that you may end up establishing a pattern that's difficult to reverse.

- Don't put your baby to sleep with a formula- or milk-filled bottle. This habit can lead to teeth problems later on.

Crying

You may as well face it — babies cry. It's their main way of expressing themselves. During the first week of life, some babies hardly cry at all; they seem so incredibly happy and peaceful. But by the second week they

☺ ☹ ☹ ☺ ☺ ☹ ☺ ☺ ☹ ☺ ☺ ☹ ☺ ☺ ☹ ☺ ☺ ☹ ☹ ☺

can turn into the loudest criers in the world. Many newborns develop a variety of crying patterns and sounds, each of which can mean a different thing. You soon learn to distinguish your baby's messages, but occasionally, a baby may cry for no apparent reason whatsoever. You can try any number of soothing techniques — walking the baby around a bit, rocking, talking, bouncing on your knee, whatever. If nothing works, and you really can't identify any problem, don't jump to the conclusion that you are a terrible parent. You aren't. Babies don't always cry for a reason, and maybe your baby just needs to cry a little!

In most cases, you can use your own common sense to figure out how to calm your crying baby. But it may help at first to have a list of all the tried-and-true strategies:

❀ Feed your baby.

❀ Burp your baby, trying various techniques.

❀ Change the diaper.

❀ Hold your baby in a warm, supportive, loving manner.

❀ Rock your baby, walk around with your baby, or change his or her position.

❀ Take your baby for a walk in the stroller or a ride in the car.

❀ Put your baby in the infant car seat and set the car seat on top of a running washing machine, holding on to it to make absolutely sure that it doesn't fall off. Some babies find the gentle shaking motion soothing.

❀ Give your baby a pacifier.

❀ Entertain your baby with a toy.

❀ Play music.

❀ Give your baby a bath.

❀ Let your baby rest and relax in a quiet room (quiet except for the sound of his or her crying, that is).

❀ Put your baby down in his or her crib to rest.

❀ Rock your baby in a baby swing — making sure that he or she is carefully strapped in and never left unattended.

❀ If all else fails, and you're assured that your baby seems not to be suffering any real discomfort, you may need to just let him or her cry! Then the trick is to find a way not to let it bother you. (Hint: Try turning up the radio.)

C is for colic

Unfortunately, there is such a thing as *colic*. It is traditionally defined as a baby who cries for more than three hours a day, three days a week, for three consecutive weeks. Doctors don't know the exact cause, but some think it may be related to intestinal discomfort. Colic often starts at about 4 to 6 weeks and ends by about 12 weeks. When your baby has colic, he or she cries and cries, and little that can be done to console him or her. If you are working outside the home, and this is the time of day when you finally get to be with your baby, you may think that your baby doesn't like you. Be assured that the timing doesn't hinge on you – it's just that the evening hours are the bewitching hours. Talk to your pediatrician if your baby experiences colic.

Part 4

Caring for Your Baby and You

Caring for a newborn is the most important — and perhaps the hardest — job in the world. Your lovely little baby depends on you for food, comfort, and love. And how you spend the first year with your child makes a big difference in your child's mental and physical development.

This part shows you how to care for your newborn. You also find advice for looking after yourself and recovering from your pregnancy; after your baby's taken care of, you need to take time to think about you.

Chapter 10

Dinnertime! Feeding Your Baby

One of the first big decisions new parents make is whether to breast-feed their infants or use formula and bottles. Although the majority of parents these days choose to breast-feed, the decision is by no means an easy one. If you have difficulty deciding, take comfort in the fact that both choices are sound and legitimate. This chapter lays out the basic first steps you need, no matter which way you go.

All about Breast-Feeding

Ask almost anyone — your obstetrician, your pediatrician, your friends, total strangers — and they will advise you to breast-feed. This opinion represents, in part, a return to early 19th-century values, but also incorporates recent medical knowledge. Bottle-feeding became all the rage in the 1950s, during the peak of the baby boom, when techniques were developed to pasteurize and store cow's milk in formulas appropriate for infant nutrition. Today, breast-feeding has regained popularity largely because people and organizations such as the American College of Obstetrics and Gynecology and the American Academy of Pediatrics have come to recognize the many sound medical reasons to do it. It strengthens the baby's immune system and helps prevent allergies, asthma, and sudden infant death syndrome.

However, the decision isn't always simply a medical one. It also involves issues of convenience, aesthetics, body image, and even conditions surrounding delivery. Some women find that they are uncomfortable with the whole physical concept of breast-feeding. Others want to bottle-feed so

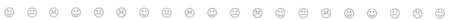
that they aren't the only one who can feed the baby. Still others have work or time pressures that make bottle-feeding more convenient. In the final analysis, the decision about how to feed the baby is a personal one that every mother has a right to decide for herself. Learning to breast-feed takes an incredible commitment, and you shouldn't feel pressured to do it if your heart isn't in it. If you have decided that bottle-feeding is the best decision for you and your baby, don't feel guilty about it.

Pros and cons of breast-feeding

Both bottle-feeding and breast-feeding have their benefits. The following two lists give you food for thought when making your feeding decision. First, some reasons to breast-feed:

* Human breast milk can strengthen the baby's immune system and help prevent allergies, asthma, and sudden infant death syndrome. It can also decrease the number of upper respiratory infections in the baby's first year of life.

* Mother's milk contains nutrients that are ideally suited to a baby's digestive system. Formula is not as easily digested, and the nutrients it contains are not as readily used by the baby.

* Human milk also contains substances that help protect a baby from infections until his or her own immune system matures. These substances are especially plentiful in the *colostrum* — the yellowish pre-milk substance that mothers' breasts secrete during the first few days after the baby is born. Colostrum has a higher protein and lower fat content than milk and contains those all-important antibodies from your immune system.

* Babies are more likely to have an allergic reaction to formula than to mother's milk.

* Breast-feeding is emotionally rewarding. Many women feel that they develop a special bond with their babies when they breast-feed, and they enjoy the closeness surrounding the whole experience.

* Breast-feeding is convenient. You can't leave home without it. You never have to carry bottles or formula with you.

* Mother's milk is cheaper than formula and bottles.

* You don't have to warm up breast milk; it's always the perfect temperature.

* Lactation (milk production) causes you to burn extra calories, which may help you lose some of the weight you gained during pregnancy.

- A breast-fed baby's bowel movements don't have as strong an odor as those babies who formula-feed.

- Breast milk is organic — no additives, no preservatives.

- Some studies suggest that women who breast-feed may reduce their lifetime risk of breast cancer.

Now, the cons of breast-feeding:

- You may not want to breast-feed. If your heart's not in it, it ain't gonna happen. Too much trial and error is involved in making breast-feeding work for someone who's not truly committed to succeeding.

- If you've tried breast-feeding and your breasts don't produce enough milk to feed your baby (or babies!), you'll have to supplement with formula.

- Breast-feeding may not fit your lifestyle. Although many working mothers are able to breast-feed, many feel that juggling the requirements of their job with those of breast-feeding is just too difficult. Bottle-feeding is one solution.

- Some women find the whole concept of feeding their baby a "bodily secretion" unpleasant.

- Breast-feeding doesn't allow other family members (or caregivers) to feed the baby.

- If you have a chronic infection — HIV, for example — you shouldn't breast-feed. Instead, bottle-feeding helps ensure that diseases aren't passed to the baby.

  One exception is women who carry the hepatitis B virus, who are able to breast-feed as long as the baby has received HBIG and the hepatitis B vaccine.

- Illness after you deliver may not allow you to breast-feed.

- Breast-feeding may not be possible (you may not be able to lactate) if you've had previous surgery on your breasts.

- If you take certain medications, you probably shouldn't breast-feed.

 In any case, if you have made an informed choice about whether to breast-feed or bottle-feed, don't let anyone make you feel guilty about your decision.

☺ ☺ ☹ ☺ ☺ ☹ ☺ ☺ ☹ ☺ ☺ ☹ ☺ ☺ ☹ ☺ ☺ ☺ ☹ ☺

Inverted nipples

Some women have inverted nipples and worry during pregnancy that their nipples will make breast-feeding difficult. Usually, the problem corrects itself before the baby is born, but a few techniques can help things along:

☀ Use the thumb and forefinger on one hand to push back the skin around the areola. If this technique doesn't bring the nipple out, use your other thumb and forefinger to gently grasp your nipple, pull it outward, and hold it for a few minutes. You can do this exercise several times a day.

☀ You can also try wearing special plastic breast cups (available at most drug stores) designed to help draw out the nipple over time.

The best idea is to start one of these preparation techniques for short sessions during the second trimester and then gradually increase the amount of time you work your nipples or wear the cups until your nipples stay out on their own.

Breast-feeding positions

If you choose to breast-feed, there's no reason why you can't get started immediately after delivery, wherever you happen to be — the birthing room, the delivery room, or the recovery room. As soon as the nurses have checked your baby's health and your baby has settled down a bit, you can begin. Things are likely to be a little awkward at first, and you may as well anticipate this situation and try not to get too frustrated. Many babies don't want to breast-feed immediately. Have patience — you and your baby will eventually get the hang of it.

You can breast-feed in one of three basic positions, as shown in Figure 10-1. Use whichever position works and is comfortable for you and your baby. Most women alternate among the positions according to where they are when they're breast-feeding.

✿ **Cradling:** The simplest way is to cradle your baby in your arms with his head next to the bend in your elbow and tilted a bit in toward your breast.

✿ **Lying down:** In the lying down position, you lie on your side in bed with the baby next to you. Support the baby with either your lower arm or pillows so that her mouth is next to your lower breast, and use your other arm to guide your baby's mouth to the nipple. This position is best for middle-of-the-night feedings or after a cesarean delivery when sitting up is still uncomfortable.

✿ **Football hold:** You cradle your baby's head in the palm of your hand and support the body with your forearm. You may find that placing a pillow underneath your arm for extra support helps in this position. You can use your free hand to hold your breast close to the baby's mouth.

☺ ☺ ☹ ☺ ☺ ☹ ☺ ☺ ☹ ☺ ☺ ☹ ☺ ☺ ☹ ☺ ☺ ☹ ☺

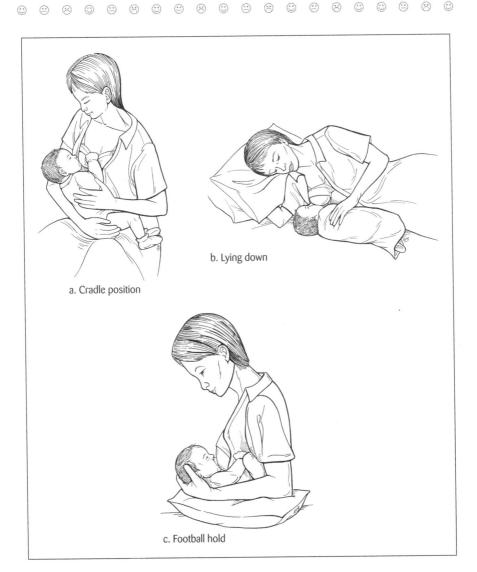

a. Cradle position

b. Lying down

c. Football hold

Figure 10-1: The three basic positions for breast-feeding.

Getting the baby to latch on

Babies are born with a suckling reflex, but many of them don't follow it enthusiastically right off the bat. Sometimes babies need some coaxing to latch onto the breast. After you have your baby in one of the basic breast-feeding positions (see the preceding section), use your nipple to gently stroke the baby's lips or cheek. This action probably causes the baby to open his mouth. If your baby doesn't seem to want to open his mouth, try

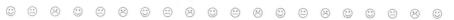
expressing (gently pressing out) a little milk — colostrum, really — and rubbing some on the baby's lips. When the mouth is wide open, bring the baby's head to your breast and gently place the baby's mouth over your entire nipple. This prodding usually causes the baby to start sucking. Make sure that the entire areola is inside the baby's mouth, because if it isn't, baby doesn't get enough milk, and you get sore nipples. However, don't stuff your breast into your baby's mouth. Rather, bring the mouth to your nipple, and let the infant take in the breast.

The tip of the baby's nose should be barely touching the skin around your breast. The only way the baby can breathe is through her nose, so be careful not to completely cover the baby's nose with your breast. If your breast obstructs the baby's nose, use your free hand to depress your breast in front of the nose to let some air in.

Feeding sessions

After your baby latches on, you know that she is sucking when you see regular, rhythmic movements of the cheeks and chin. Several minutes of sucking may go by before your milk letdown occurs.

If your baby stops sucking without letting go of the nipple, insert your finger into the corner of his mouth to break the suction. (If you just pull your breast straight out, you'll end up with sore nipples.)

When switching from one breast to the other, stop to burp your baby by laying her either over your shoulder or your lap and gently patting her back. You should burp her again when the feeding is finished.

Typically, mothers breast-feed eight to twelve times a day (averaging ten). This pattern enables your body to produce an optimal amount of milk, and it allows your baby to get the proper amount of nutrition for healthy growth and development. Try to space the feedings fairly evenly throughout the day; of course, your baby has some influence on the schedule. You don't have to wake your baby for a feeding — unless your pediatrician specifically advises you to do so. You especially don't have to wake your baby at night; if the baby's willing to sleep through, just count yourself lucky.

You can tell whether your baby is getting enough milk by watching for the following indications:

* Your baby nurses ten times a day on average.

* Your baby gains weight.

* Your baby has six to eight wet diapers a day.

❁ Your baby has two to three bowel movements a day.

❁ Your baby's urine is pale yellow (not dark and concentrated).

Breast-feeding diet

During breast-feeding, as during pregnancy, your nutrition is largely a matter of educated common sense. The quality of your breast milk isn't significantly affected by your diet unless your eating habits are truly inadequate. However, if you don't take in enough calories, your body has a difficult time producing adequate milk.

When you're breast-feeding, you should take in an extra 400 to 600 calories a day over and above what you would normally eat. The exact amount varies, of course, according to how much you weigh and how much fat you gained during pregnancy. Because lactating does burn fat, breast-feeding is a good way to help get rid of some of the extra fat stores you may have. But avoid losing weight too fast, or your milk production will suffer. Also, avoid gaining weight while you're breast-feeding. If you find that you're putting on more pounds, you're most likely taking in too many calories.

In addition to calories, you also need extra vitamins and minerals — especially vitamin D, calcium, and iron. Keep taking your prenatal vitamins or some other balanced supplement while you're nursing. Also consume extra calcium — either a supplement or extra servings of milk, yogurt, and other dairy products.

Breast milk is mainly water (87 percent). To produce plenty of breast milk, you must take in at least 72 extra ounces of fluid per day, which is about nine extra glasses of milk, juice, or water. Don't go overboard, however, because if you drink too many fluids, your milk production may actually decrease.

Problems that breast-feeding mothers may face

One of the greatest misconceptions about breast-feeding is that it comes easily and naturally to everyone. In fact, breast-feeding takes learning and practice. Problems can range from a little nipple soreness to, in rare cases, infections in the milk ducts. This section discusses breast-feeding problems that some women experience.

Sore nipples

Many women experience some temporary nipple soreness during the first few days that they breast-feed. Fortunately, for most women, the pain is

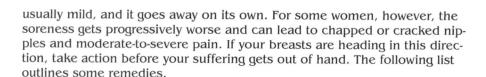
usually mild, and it goes away on its own. For some women, however, the soreness gets progressively worse and can lead to chapped or cracked nipples and moderate-to-severe pain. If your breasts are heading in this direction, take action before your suffering gets out of hand. The following list outlines some remedies.

❋ Review your breast-feeding technique to make sure that your baby is positioned correctly. If the baby isn't getting the entire nipple and areola in his or her mouth, the soreness is likely to continue. Try changing the baby's position slightly with each feeding.

❋ Increase the number of feedings and feed for less time at each feeding. This way, your baby won't be as hungry and may not suck as hard.

❋ Definitely continue to feed on the sore breast, even if only for a few minutes. This feeding is important to keep the nipple conditioned to nursing. If you let it heal completely, the soreness will only start all over again when you feed from that nipple again. Have your baby feed on the least sore breast first, because that's when your baby's sucking is most vigorous.

❋ Express a little breast milk manually before you put the baby to the breast. This action helps initiate the letdown reflex so that the baby doesn't have to suck as long and hard to achieve letdown.

❋ Don't use any irritating chemicals or soaps on your nipples.

❋ After your baby finishes feeding, don't wipe off your nipples. Let them air-dry for as long as possible. Wiping them with a cloth may cause needless irritation.

❋ Exposing the nipples to air helps to toughen the skin, so try to walk around the house with your nipples exposed as much as possible. Also, if you wear a nursing bra, try leaving the flaps down as you go about your business at your house. As the fabric from your clothes rubs against them, your nipples toughen.

❋ If you're using pads to soak up leakage from your breasts, change them as soon as they get moist, or they may chafe your nipples.

❋ Try massaging vitamin E oil, ointment, olive oil, or lanolin into sore nipples and then letting them air dry (wipe off any excess before breastfeeding). It may sound kind of silly, but an old product called Udder Cream or Bag Balm, which was developed to treat chapped teats on milk cows, has found new popularity among some breast-feeding women. In fact, many drug stores and cosmetics stores now sell the cream. It contains lanolin and may be of help, if you can deal with the bovine name.

❋ Apply dry (not moist) and warm (not hot) heat to the nipples several times a day. You can use a hot water bottle filled with warm water.

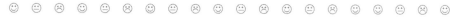

Engorgement

When the breasts become engorged with milk, they can hurt. One way to avoid painful engorgement is to begin breast-feeding right after the baby is born. Other strategies that help include wearing a firm but not tight bra and massaging the breasts before feeding. Massaging facilitates letdown and relieves some of the engorgement. You can also try placing warm compresses on your breasts. (Some women feel that ice packs work better — try both and see which works best for you.)

Clogged ducts

Sometimes, some of the milk ducts in the breast may become clogged with debris. If this happens, a small, firm, red lump may form inside the breast. The lump may be tender, but it's usually not associated with a fever or excruciating pain. The best way to treat a clogged breast duct is to try to completely empty that breast after each feeding. Start the baby out on that breast when he or she is most hungry. If the baby doesn't completely empty the breast, use a breast pump on that side until all the milk is drained. Also, applying heat to the lump and massaging it manually is helpful. Most important, keep feeding!

Mastitis (breast infection)

Breast infections (mastitis) are reasonably common — occurring in about 2 percent of all breast-feeding women. They are usually caused by bacteria that come from the baby's mouth. The symptoms of mastitis include a warm, hard, red breast; high fever (usually over 101°); and malaise (like when you have the flu and your whole body feels achy). Infections are most likely to happen two to four weeks after delivery, but they can occur earlier or later than that. If these symptoms develop, call your doctor immediately.

Bottle-Feeding for Beginners

Suppose you've decided to forego breast-feeding in favor of formula. Or you've been breast-feeding for a number of weeks or months, and you want to switch. This section tells you what you need to know to get your baby started on bottles.

Stopping milk production

If you do decide to formula-feed, you need to stop the process of milk production in your breasts. Milk production is triggered by warmth and breast stimulation. So to stop the production of milk, you want to create the opposite environment. Here are some suggestions:

❀ Wear a tight-fitting bra.

❀ Apply ice packs to your breasts when they become engorged. This engorgement generally happens around the third or fourth day after your baby is born.

☺ ☹ ☹ ☺ ☺ ☹ ☺ ☺ ☹ ☺ ☺ ☹ ☺ ☺ ☹ ☺ ☺ ☺ ☹ ☺

❋ Keep ice packs inside your bra, or use small packages of frozen vegetables, like peas or corn, which you can easily fold to fit within a
   bra. (You probably don't want to go out in public this way, though.)

❋ Place cold cabbage leaves inside your bra. Cabbage works chemi-
   cally to reduce the production of milk.

❋ Let cold water run over your breasts during a shower.

If you are going to breast-feed for a short period of time (6 to 12 weeks),
consider giving your baby one bottle of formula per day while you are nursing to help make the transition easier.

Bottle-feeding basics

The most common position for bottle-feeding your baby is to hold the baby
cradled in one arm, close to your body. You will find it most comfortable
to put a pillow on your lap, which eases the strain on your arms and neck.
Most women find it easier to always hold the baby in the same arm and
in the same direction. For example, if you are right-handed, you may want
to hold your baby in your left arm, and the bottle in the right. When the
baby is a little older and has better control of his or her head and neck
muscles, you may want to lay the baby in front of you vertically along your
legs for a change of pace. This way, the baby can look straight ahead at
you, and you both can make eye contact.

Pediatricians generally don't recommend propping up a baby's bottle by
laying it on a pillow next to the baby's mouth, because propping implies that
the baby is being left unattended. Also, a baby lying flat on his or her back
with the bottle propped creates more potential for choking. Propping a bottle
may also promote tooth decay.

Many parents are told to sterilize bottles by boiling them in water, but most
pediatricians think that this step is unnecessary. After all, a mother who
breast-feeds doesn't have to boil her nipples!

Many parents choose to warm their baby's bottle, but heating it isn't
necessary. You can warm a bottle in different ways. You can place the
bottle in a container filled with hot water or use a bottle warmer.

If you use the microwave to heat your baby's bottle, be careful. The formula
may heat unevenly, and some parts of it may be too hot for the baby.
However, if you shake the bottle after warming it, it may be okay. Just make
sure you first shake some onto your wrist (which is more sensitive than your
hand) to check the temperature.

☺ ☺ ☹ ☺ ☺ ☹ ☺ ☺ ☹ ☺ ☺ ☹ ☺ ☺ ☹ ☺ ☺ ☺ ☹ ☺

Saving leftover formula is generally not a good idea. However, some pediatricians say that reusing a bottle once is okay, so talk it over with your baby's doctor. In any case, don't leave a bottle filled with formula sitting outside the refrigerator for longer than an hour because warmth encourages the growth of bacteria that can upset your baby's stomach.

Here are some other tips:

❀ **Don't swaddle the baby too much or keep him too warm during feeding.** The baby may get so comfortable that he falls asleep instead of feeding.

❀ **Change the baby's diaper in the middle of a feeding.** This may help to wake her up, so that she can finish the rest of the bottle.

❀ **If your baby has trouble finding the nipple to put in his mouth,** stroke his cheek, and he will turn in that direction.

❀ **To check to see whether the baby is hungry,** put the tip of your finger (a clean finger) into her mouth to see whether she starts to suck.

❀ **Keep the bottle tilted in such a way as to completely fill the nipple with the formula,** thereby minimizing the amount of air that gets into the baby.

Chapter **11**

Playtime and Bedtime and Every Time in Between

This chapter looks into the three day-to-day tasks that every parent needs to know about — bathing your baby, changing diapers, and putting your baby to sleep.

Most parents agree that getting the baby to sleep is the hardest one. As this chapter explains, babies' sleep patterns change as they grow older, and recognizing and accommodating these changing patterns are two of the most difficult tasks parents have. Hang in there. When your child is a teenager and you have trouble rousting him or her out of bed, you'll actually feel nostalgic for the old days when your child woke up every morning at 6 o'clock sharp.

Bathing Babies

Giving your baby a bath three or four times a day isn't necessary, even though she may look like she needs one after every meal. Parents tend to give a lot of baths because freshly washed kids smell so good. Babies between the ages of 3 months to 1 year need a bath once a day or at least every other day if that's all you can manage (Chapter 9 explains how to bathe a newborn). Don't spare that washcloth on the face and hands during the day, especially after meals. The little ones tend to fight you on the face washing, but remember that you're the boss.

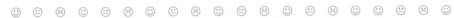

Washing a baby boy

A baby boy's circumcised penis requires special care until the circumcision has healed. Follow your doctor's instructions, which usually include placing a petroleum jelly gauze on the tip of the penis and replacing it when you change diapers. The petroleum jelly prevents the tip of the penis from sticking to the diaper. Once it heals, you can stop using the petroleum jelly. If a plastic bell was used to circumcise your baby, you can expect it to fall off on its own in seven to ten days. Because there are now different kinds of devices for the circumcising process, get specific instructions from your doctor about proper care.

A circumcised penis will be red and may develop a yellowish tissue as it heals. Call your doctor if your baby has fever, or pus is draining from the circumcision site.

If your baby is not circumcised, no special care is required. You may occasionally notice whitish lumps of matter called *smegma* coming from underneath your child's foreskin. This is normal and is just the shedding of old skin cells that work their way out from under the foreskin. Also remember that you do not want to force back the foreskin in an uncircumcised infant.

 You should always have one hand on your baby when she bathes. She'll squirm and topple over easily, and if you pour water over her face she'll stiffen her little body and fall backward. If you aren't holding her well, she'll bonk her head. Baby stores sell some wondrous contraptions that are supposed to help hold up your baby while you bathe her. Save your money. Just do a good job supporting her with your arms and hands and only fill the tub with an inch or two of water.

Changing a Diaper Step-By-Step

Changing a diaper well is an art form — a delicate procedure that deals with sensitive body parts, and a messy procedure that requires special tools and equipment and the mobility of a master acrobatics instructor. This section explains how to change a diaper and what to do about diaper rash.

Changing soiled diapers

Many sore baby bottoms result because a baby isn't cleaned properly, and the poor baby suffers. To become a top-notch diaper changer, following these instructions:

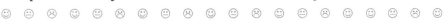
1 Open and unfold the new diaper.

Lay your baby (wearing a used diaper) on top of the new diaper and hand your baby a toy or make sure a mobile is hanging over the baby's head (this is the distraction so baby won't try to escape).

2 Unfasten the used diaper.

If you're changing a boy baby, open the diaper just a little bit at first, because air tends to make junior want to go right then and there; with the angle of the baby lying down, you may get sprayed in the face. Alternately, you can also open the diaper and lay a washcloth or cloth diaper across the baby's penis as a shield.

3 Gather your baby's feet with one hand and lift with the other.

Remove the dirty diaper, wad it up, and — if it was his or her turn to do this — toss it at your spouse. Otherwise, dispose of it.

4 Clean your baby's bottom.

After your baby's bottom is clean, lower your baby onto the clean diaper.

5 Fasten the diaper on your baby.

Say something cute: Your baby will smile and prepare to soil the diaper again.

6 Wash your hands thoroughly.

You don't want to spread hidden poop or germs around.

 Newborns experience an insecure feeling when their diapers are changed. That is why they appear cranky, cry, and reach their arms out to the side. Help your baby feel a little more secure by keeping either one of your hands or a blanket or towel on his or her stomach for as long as possible. This pressure helps calm your baby.

 When changing your little girl's diaper, wipe her bottom from front to back. Doing so helps avoid any kind of bladder or urinary tract infections from the bacteria being spread.

Winning the diaper battle

You can handle those difficult diaper changes by keeping a stash of toys or interesting objects close at hand so that when you lay your little baby down for a diaper change you'll have something to keep those idle hands busy. You can also hang a mobile over the table.

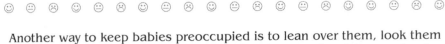

Another way to keep babies preoccupied is to lean over them, look them in the eye, and sing or talk to them. Doing the occasional *tummy tzerbert* also preoccupies babies. To do this, place your lips on baby's tummy and blow out to make a *bpbpbpb* sound.

When your baby wakes up in the middle of the night, wait to change his diaper until he's half through with the feeding (either half the bottle, or done with one breast if breast-feeding). That way you'll satisfy your baby's hunger right away, and you won't have to wake him up to change a diaper after the little one has dozed off to sleep.

Dealing with diaper rash

Diaper rash results from dirty diapers being left on too long and from gastrointestinal problems. A rash also can develop because of poop that's acidic — because of a stomach virus, teething, or something your child ate that was too strong for his or her system (such as citrus foods for babies younger than 1 year old). In any case, this kind of bowel movement can instantly cause a rash that may resemble little blisters. Table 11-1 explains all the reasons for a diaper rash and the different ways to fix the problem.

Table 11-1 Diaper Rash

Situation	Solution
Allergy to the type of diaper you're using	Change diaper brands.
Allergy to the type of baby wipe you're using	Change baby wipe brands or just use soap and water. Try unscented wipes.
Detergent used for cloth diapers is too strong	Change detergent to one without perfume or dyes.
A wet or dirty diaper is left on too long	Check your child's diaper often.
Hot weather	Your baby's sweat, combined with urine and bowel movements, and mixed with a diaper bottom that's warm, dark, and wet begs for diaper rash to occur. This is a good time to go diaperless for short periods of time.
Consistent diarrhea	Diarrhea can be caused from teething, a stomach virus, tension, drinking too much juice, a food allergy, or eating something that's too strong for a child's system.
Food sensitivity	Change formulas, or take your child off the solid food recently started. Diaper rash can be a sign of your child reacting to a new food.

Important baby bag contents

As your baby grows older, you'll find that you have less to carry with you. And, if your trips are short, you don't necessarily have to load up with everything. But here is a list of things you don't want to be caught without.

- Baby wipes
- Bib
- Blanket
- Bottles
- Burp-up towel
- Change of clothing

- Changing cushion
- Diaper-rash ointment and baby Tylenol
- Diapers
- Food/spoon/ snack
- Nipples

- Pacifier
- Water
- Doctor's phone number
- Insurance and allergy information

A baby's dirty diaper needs to be changed immediately. The combination of the moisture from the diaper and the lack of air to dry it out causes rashes and chafing.

 The best way to take care of diaper rash is not to use baby wipes, but, instead, wash the baby's bottom off in a sink with warm, soapy water. Baby wipes are soapy and may irritate the rash. Pat the bottom dry and apply a zinc-oxide ointment. If the rash lasts more than three days, contact your doctor, who'll likely prescribe an industrial-strength ointment that'll clear it up pronto.

Exposing rash-prone areas to the air for a while helps prevent diaper rash and clear up rashes that already have started. After changing the diaper, washing off the area, and patting it dry, allow your baby to crawl or walk around without the diaper for some time. Don't put diaper rash ointment on a baby who's walking around bottomless (the ointment will get everywhere!).

Rock-a-Bye Baby: Getting Your Infant to Sleep

If only all kids would sleep as easily and soundly as a newborn, your life as parents would be near perfect. Of course, keeping them asleep for any amount of time is the trick.

☺ ☺ ☹ ☺ ☺ ☺ ☹ ☺ ☺ ☹ ☺ ☺ ☹ ☺ ☺ ☹ ☺ ☺ ☺ ☹ ☺

Developing a sleeping routine for babies varies from child to child. The child's temperament and family's lifestyle determine how he or she sleeps. Coming up with a sleeping schedule is always a challenge. Be open to different approaches to getting babies to sleep, bearing in mind that not all methods will work with your baby.

Baby sleep facts

Babies have shorter and lighter sleep cycles than adults. That is why they usually wake up two or three times a night from birth to 6 months. As they grow older, they wake up once or twice a night from 6 months to 1 year; and then they may awaken once a night when they reach 1 to 2 years of age.

Babies' sleep habits typically are developed by their individual temperaments rather than your abilities to get your baby to sleep. It isn't your fault that your baby wakes up, but your before-bedtime rituals do have something to do with how easily your child goes to bed. Even when you're dead tired and need to sleep, you can't force your baby to go to sleep. You can, however, create a safe environment that enables your baby to fall asleep easily. Doing so is the best way to establish long-term healthy sleep habits.

Helping your baby sleep

Creating a safe and comfortable environment for your child makes falling asleep much easier. Some things that you can do to help your baby fall asleep include:

❋ **Hold your baby often during the day.** Babies love to be held close, such as in a baby sling.

❋ **Keep your baby on as much of a regular schedule as possible,** such as regular feeding times and bedtimes. You also need to consider how late naps may keep babies up later at night.

❋ **Establish a relaxed, quiet routine leading up to bedtime,** such as a warm bath or massage, singing, or reading a book. Rock your baby. Nurse the baby at your breast or with a bottle. Any active play primes your baby, meaning that she'll be more likely to stay awake.

❋ **Wait until your baby has entered a deep sleep (you'll notice the limp limbs and a motionless face) before moving your baby to a cradle or bed.** However, when babies turn 5 to 6 months old, start putting your baby in the crib when she starts getting sleepy. That helps your baby associate the crib with the time to go to sleep.

❋ **Wrap your newborn with the blanket the way they do in hospitals.** Newborns prefer to be *swaddled* in this way. Older babies, however, usually prefer loose covers.

❀ **Playing a soothing sound,** such as a recording of a mother's heartbeat, sounds of a water fall, ocean sounds, or soft background noise like a fan or dishwasher.

Rituals

Whatever ritual or habit you start with your newborn to get her to sleep is the same ritual or habit she'll come to expect as she gets older. So start your child's lifetime sleeping habits off right. Lay your baby down in her bed when it's time for her to sleep — meaning after your child has eaten and when you see her going into that deep sleep stage. When your child gets older, she'll understand that lying in her bed means sleep time.

The older your children get, the less they'll sleep, and the more their personalities will come out. Then they start exerting their will — and everything is messy from then on. Be grateful for your newborn — she typically doesn't need help falling asleep.

Bedtime

Babies actually adapt to schedules rather nicely. Always allow room for changes in these schedules. As they grow, their naps grow shorter, and they sleep longer during the night. Basically, as much as parents hate it, they grow up. They're heading for that day when they won't need naps.

Getting your older kids to bed is easier when they have a set schedule. These schedules slowly change over time, so you must be aware of and sensitive to these changes as they happen.

Establish a bedtime for your kids. Remember, this is your *child's* bedtime. It's the time when she acts like she needs to go to bed. It isn't the time when *you* would like her to go to bed. Those are usually two different times. Your child's bedtime also isn't the time that you think she ought to go to bed, simply because that's when you went to bed when you were a kid. Your children have their own clocks to go by. And, when you have more than one child, be aware that each of your children has an individual bedtime, depending on his or her age.

You have to be observant of your child to determine what his needs are. Pay attention to how long his naps are and how long he sleeps through the night. When you're aware of your child's sleeping patterns, predicting when he needs to go to bed becomes easier.

Chapter 12

Happiness Is . . . a Routine?

Whether your child reaches his or her potential depends on how much intellectual and sensory stimulation your child receives during the first five years of life. Babies need stimulation for their brains to develop and for them to become well-rounded kids. In other words, your child's surroundings influence how intelligent and well-adjusted your child grows to be. This chapter presents some ideas to launch your baby in a smart direction.

The Importance of Play and Stimulation

The way you bring up your infant actually determines how the brain grows. One-hundred billion brain cells called *neurons* lurk inside your newborn's noodle. These miniscule cells like to move and connect with each other. The bridges they form create wiring that enables your baby to process information and experience the world through the senses. More connections mean a smarter kid, and stimulating a baby is what causes these neurons to get together. The sounds, colors, smells, and touches you provide trigger new and improved circuitry inside your baby's brain.

 Every time you wiggle her fingers, rock your baby to sleep with a lullaby, sprinkle water on your baby's tummy during bath time, and act silly, you stimulate more brain cells to form vibrant new pathways. And when you decorate your child's surroundings and supply different ways to play, you cause actions and reactions that prompt additional brain bridges.

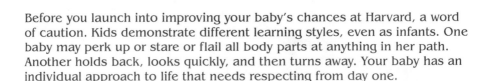

Before you launch into improving your baby's chances at Harvard, a word of caution. Kids demonstrate different learning styles, even as infants. One baby may perk up or stare or flail all body parts at anything in her path. Another holds back, looks quickly, and then turns away. Your baby has an individual approach to life that needs respecting from day one.

Most kids follow the same basic developmental path. But some take their time, while others whiz through each stage or speed along and plateau at different rest stops. And many kids exhibit uneven mental and physical progress. The schedule your child is on provides another sign of your infant's uniqueness.

Table 12-1 gives you some general milestones you can expect from your infant, the child from 0 to 12 months old. These are just guidelines, not hard-and-fast rules of developmental conduct.

Table 12-1 A Baby's First Year

	Newborn	*3 to 6 Months*	*9 to 12 Months*
Language	Follows sounds, cries when uncomfortable, startles at loud sounds	Differentiates cries, imitates sounds and syllables, laughs aloud, babbles, shakes head "no"	Understands words, says first words, waves "bye-bye"
Senses and motor	Tracks moving objects, hears well, lifts head, flails all body parts, sees best at 10 inches, sucks, yawns	Grasps and holds, sits independently, rolls from stomach to back, explores with mouth, holds rattle	Uses spoon, feeds with fingers, crawls, takes first steps, bangs objects, makes objects disappear
Social and mental	Smiles, quiets down with comforting, recognizes sight and smell of parents	Says "no" without understanding, reaches toward caregiver, shows interest in surroundings, recognizes toys or bottle	Begins to understand routines, connects with parents, cries when parents leave, sometimes stops at "no"

Bringing the World to Your Baby

Because young babies can't move anywhere, you have to bring the world to them. Your role during the first few months of life is to provide items to play with (besides yourself, of course). These objects titillate the senses of touch, sight, hearing, and smell.

144

Toys that foster learning

The quest for the perfect toy, more specifically the perfect learning toy, is way overblown. Don't believe the hype about "jumpstarting" your child's learning at two weeks or advertisements that scream, "Genius in the making." Sure, expensive, pretty toys brighten a baby's room, but you don't have to buy those sorts of toys. Your baby doesn't care how much you spend, at least not now. Your baby is just as happy with a ball of aluminum foil on a string as he or she is with a fancy, expensive mobile. You baby's enthusiasm for simple fun stuff lasts for years.

Baby brain games

You want some inexpensive, yet worthwhile, games to play with your infant? Can't get much simpler than these:

❀ **Play music, any kind that suits you, and make sounds for your baby to track.** Clap your hands, snap your fingers, and utter unusual sound effects in different positions around your infant's head, while she lays on her back or stomach.

❀ **Hold a bright-colored ball or toy in front of your baby to track the object as you move it.** By about 8 to 10 weeks, encourage your bundle of joy to reach for the object.

❀ **Hang a safety mirror over the crib so she can see herself.** As she gets older, make sure a tall mirror is fastened to a door to give her a good look at how she plays.

❀ **Draw line art of a face on cardboard and tuck it into your baby's infant seat or the side of the crib.** Babies respond to simple patterns. They get most excited by faces. Even a no-talent-needed happy face on a piece of rectangular cardboard tucked in a car seat can do the job.

❀ **Offer familiar but safe household objects to babies 3 to 6 months and older who love to explore with their hands.** Nothing fancy here. Think about plastic and metal bowls and bottles, measuring cups and spoons, which are favorites, along with keys, clothes pins (relics of the past), and swatches of bright non-fuzzy cloth that won't come off in her mouth. Consider, too, frozen teething rings to gnaw on while in the throws of painful teething, wooden spoons to bang, empty cardboard boxes for your crawler, and paper bags to shake objects in and out. And keep in mind that for the first year or two, gift wrap is much more exciting as a toy than the gift(s) inside.

❀ **Cut the toes off brightly-colored baby socks and put one on each hand.** Your baby will have hours of fun wiggling her fingers and focusing on her colored hand.

Offering Different Points of View

You can't see much lying on your back, and your baby isn't ready to sit up, even with support, until between 4 and 6 months. So you need to provide different points of view, as follows:

❀ **Lean your infant in your lap while you sit.**

❀ **Swing her in an automated swing.** Besides providing a different height perspective, a swing calms babies long enough for you to finish dinner or an important conversation. Some swings come with battery-operated music boxes, a definite improvement over the crank type that needs rewinding every few minutes and jolts your snoozing babe awake. If your infant is too floppy, prop her sides with rolled towels or diapers.

❀ **Lay your baby on her stomach a couple times a day.** This encourages her to lift her head and get the idea of crawling some day.

❀ **Carry your baby in a sack close to your body.** Besides your being able to talk to your child easily without snoops listening in, infants thrive on physical contact and being close to the heartbeat that sustained them for nine months in utero. For a different perspective, turn your baby around, so that he or she can watch the world as you move along.

You can buy two different types of front pouches, as pictured in Figure 12-1. Both allow your hands to be free to do other things. A sling works best for newborns, who sleep a lot. Front packs provide more support, so your baby can look around.

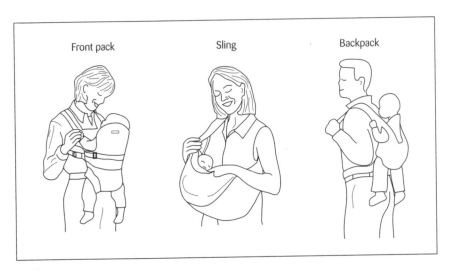

Figure 12-1: Look ma — no hands!

☺ ☺ ☹ ☺ ☺ ☹ ☺ ☺ ☹ ☺ ☺ ☹ ☺ ☺ ☹ ☺ ☺ ☹ ☺

Babies get heavy after a few months in either front carrier, so you won't use yours for long. Try to borrow a baby pouch or buy one at a resale store to use until your baby grows too heavy for you to carry kangaroo style. Because most front carriers are washable, using someone else's shouldn't be a germ problem.

✿ **Plop your baby in a backpack after her head stops bobbing.** Backpacks elevate baby, giving her the same birds-eye view that you see, and they distribute weight better, which lessens your chances of backaches and reduces your trips to the chiropractor. Some are limp, as in Figure 12-1, while others have a metal frame to support heavier babes. With either version, you may want to tie lose tendrils back. Babies grab and pull anything in their reach — it's part of the learning process.

 Unless you want your hair conditioned with soggy slobber or sticky crumbs, refrain from giving your baby nibbles while being carried in a backpack. These snacks can also cause choking, so steer clear.

✿ **Strap your baby into an infant seat.** New versions adjust for sitting and reclining or they bounce, which you can activate with your foot while busying yourself with other occupations.

Tracking Milestones

Table 12-2 is designed to help you track milestones that your developing baby will reach during his or her first six months. The first time you notice your baby doing these wonderful activities for the first time, write down the date. You can also add more at the bottom of the table.

Table 12-2 Your Baby's Milestones

Date	Activity
	Holds hands up in front of body
	Looks straight ahead
	Looks around
	On back, baby rolls from side to side
	On stomach, baby lifts head
	On stomach, baby supports him- or herself on one arm
	Baby rolls from stomach to back

continued

147

☺ ☺ ☹ ☺ ☺ ☹ ☺ ☺ ☹ ☺ ☺ ☹ ☺ ☺ ☹ ☺ ☺ ☺ ☹ ☺

Table 12-2 Your Baby's Milestones (continued)

Date	Activity
	Baby rolls into a sitting position
	Baby reaches for toys
	Baby grips toys
	Baby puts objects in his or her mouth

Giving Your Baby Exercise

Sometimes, even with the best intentions, knowing what to do all day with a newborn is difficult. Lots of books give precise instructions for manipulating your baby's body parts. But you don't need to get fancy. Use your organizational skills to come up with a schedule that incorporates everything you believe stimulates your baby's body and mind. In other words, exercise your baby!

Exercise activities make your baby's body more flexible. And the time together builds on the bond you already have. Try these exercises:

❀ Take one body part (such as the right arm) at a time and gently stretch it, move it up, move it down, cross it over to the other side of the body, and place it back down. Go to the left arm, and do the same thing. Then move on to other body parts.

❀ Turn your baby over and gently try similar exercises. Play music and keep time by moving your baby to the beat.

❀ Place your baby face-down over a large ball. Rock her up and back. As she matures, her arms will go out to protect her head. This game gives your baby a sense of her body in space.

❀ Push your baby in a swing, after she can sit without flopping.

❀ Hold and carry your baby around town. Nothing stimulates better during the first three months of life than snuggling with a parent as the world flies by.

Rub a vitamin E oil, baby oil, or other cold-pressed oil over one body part at a time. Gentle massage awakens nerve endings and the senses. Use different textured materials, such as terrycloth or velour, to evoke different sensations. Massage now can pay off later. Down the road, during times of stress, you'll be pleasantly surprised that you can calm your baby by gently rubbing a hand, a leg, her back, or her stomach. The calming memory lingers throughout the body.

Decorating Your Baby's Room

Ideally, a baby's space is more than a pretty place to sleep. The room is a total environment where your child can play, grow, and learn. It's also a place to go when the outside world closes in, when parents become unreasonable, or when your little one needs a calming or stimulating place.

 Some educators recommend keeping the room exactly the same for at least the first year. This gives your child the opportunity to feel safe while discovering new wonders at each new developmental stage. These folks also suggest that you crawl around the room to get an idea what your baby sees, hears, and feels.

Your choice of decorations, from furniture to toys to wall hangings, says a lot about what you expect for your child. The following sections give you some suggestions to help you and nature walk your baby along the developmental road.

Spending time in the crib

Babies don't always sleep. And you aren't always carrying around or interacting with your infant. So think about the following ways to enliven your baby's world and improve her brain circuitry with stimulating crib decorations.

* **Hang brightly colored pieces of cloth or paper on the sides of the crib or overhead.** Babies respond to bright colors visually and with body movements. With time, they elicit wonderful baby sounds, the beginnings of speech and language. Colorful bibs tie easily to crib slats. Inexpensive place mats, especially of animals, double as touchable, washable crib artwork.

* **Make or buy a baby mobile to string in the crib.** Remember that your baby keeps her head turned toward the side for the first six weeks. So hang the mobile to one side or the other initially. After about six weeks, your infant can focus straight up toward the ceiling and appreciate stimulation from overhead. This trains her eyes and contributes to her understanding of where objects are in relation to body parts.

☺ ☺ ☹ ☺ ☺ ☹ ☺ ☺ ☹ ☺ ☺ ☹ ☺ ☺ ☹ ☺ ☺ ☺ ☹ ☺

✱ **Consider musical mobiles.** They may be more expensive than non-musical ones, but the sounds help your baby miss you less, which translates into more time for you to do other things. Modern battery-operated music boxes also keep the auditory stimulation coming for unlimited amounts of time, soothing your baby and helping her focus her hearing and differentiate sounds.

Some educators advocate a floor bed or a mattress on the floor, turning the entire room into a giant playpen. This setup allows free exploration of the entire room after your baby begins to crawl. To keep your baby — and the rest of the house — safe with this setup, put a baby gate in the doorway. And make sure the room is baby-proofed for tiny objects that can be swallowed and heavy objects that can topple on little heads.

Going from crib to floor

Make or sew a textured mat with squares of different materials affixed to a rubber pad that you can place under your baby, either in the crib or on the floor. Each movement gives your infant another tactile experience. One square can be fuzzy, another rougher, another velvety. You get the idea.

If you have a choice for floors in your baby's room, consider indoor/outdoor rugs. They're warm, washable, and slip-proof, which is what you want as your baby starts pulling herself up to explore.

Sprucing up the walls

Hang pictures, posters, photos, or whatever you want your baby to observe. She does notice what's on the walls as you carry her around, and she begins to point at them and make sounds. These simple experiences around the house build language.

Babies particularly like pictures with lots of little objects in them to point out and name — pictures of animals and family members (not that these two categories go together). Expect your baby to first notice brightly colored images or primary colors that have plenty of *contrast*, like black or red against a white background.

Recognizing color theory

Babies love color and contrast. The brighter the better. That's why so many new toys and baby products come in black, white, and red, the colors your baby sees best until 6 months of age. High-contrast, bold colors hold your infant's attention longer, visually stimulating her to kick, wave the air, and wiggle around, usually all at once.

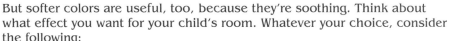

But softer colors are useful, too, because they're soothing. Think about what effect you want for your child's room. Whatever your choice, consider the following:

❁ Use washable — that means really scrubbable — paint or wallpaper only.

❁ Make nonsexist color choices. Choose a pastel because you want a soothing environment, not because your baby is a girl. All babies prefer primary colors, so don't program your girl for passivity and boy for boldness from birth because of the color of your baby's room.

Containing yourself

Plan ahead to organize your baby's room in an orderly fashion, because the room won't stay that way long after she starts moving around. But even though the room will get messy, by organizing it, you're helping your child understand how to categorize and sort objects, which enhances language development and early math skills. A bonus for you is easier cleanup.

Use boxes, plastic containers, stacking crates, and laundry baskets for different sizes of toys. As your baby matures, she can sort with you and later toss objects into their rightful places on her own.

Talking to Your Baby

The easiest and proven-most-effective way to create a child who loves learning is to talk to him. Describe to your baby what he's seeing, feeling, and experiencing. Because the ability to hear and speak language comes before understanding, your voice inflections tell your baby a lot about what you're saying. Talk to your baby to develop language, to stimulate auditory senses, and, of course, to interact with him.

❁ **Talk to your baby about his day from wakeup to final shut-eye.** Go about your regular activities and talk about them. At the store, point out fruits and vegetables. In the car, watch other cars and trucks and houses. At home, review names of different furniture, toys, and cleaning supplies.

  Use understandable, simple words in short, simple sentences, not baby talk. You want to model the type of language your child should speak as he gets older.

❁ **Point out links between real objects and pictures of objects.** Name what you call objects to provide language for the visual cues.

❁ **Create a photo scrapbook that shows important people in your child's life.** This is particularly a good idea for keeping the memory of out-of-town friends and relatives alive. But don't forget everyone in your household, too, so that you provide a framework for linking people with pictures and names.

❋ **Prepare another scrapbook of pictures of common objects in your child's life.** Photos are best because they look more like the real thing, but pictures from newspapers, magazines, catalogs, and junk-mail work, too. Kids love spending inordinate amounts of time picking out and later naming objects in their lives.

❋ **Gather more photos, this time of actions, like eating and sleeping, that your child experiences.** This type of scrapbook provides a way of developing verbs, those action words that are critical for making a complete sentence when you talk and write.

Reading to Your Baby

Reading at every stage is critical for raising a smart child. Call it snuggle time, quiet time, something-to-do together time, or whatever else works for you. Nuzzling up with your baby and a book feels good. It provides special time for baby to absorb language and pay attention without the fuss of your other must-do, scheduled activities. Regular reading lets your baby know that you care, want to spend time together, and find reading so important you schedule it every day or evening.

Reading to infants offers the bonus of presenting rhythmic patterns that the developing brain craves. Unlike everyday speech, formal writing for books often organizes *syntax* (the grammar and structure of words) so that your baby receives orderly incoming auditory information. Even though your infant can't understand the meaning of what you read, he or she gains helpful hints about how to acquire linguistic competency.

Chapter 13

The Baby's Taken Care of, Now What about Me?

According to the old adage, it takes nine months for a woman to make a baby and nine months for her body to return to normal afterwards. In reality, the time it takes to recover from childbirth varies widely from woman to woman. But most of the changes your body goes through during pregnancy revert to normal during the postpartum period, which begins immediately after delivery of the placenta and lasts for six to eight weeks.

As you go through this period of change, you're likely to have many questions about what you can do to make the postpartum transition as easy as possible. This chapter tells you what life may be like as your body gets back into its old shape, as you begin to have sex again, and as you deal with all the physical and psychological challenges of new motherhood.

Postpartum: In the Hospital

The average hospital stay after an uncomplicated vaginal delivery is 24 to 48 hours. After a cesarean, the average stay is three to four days. In some hospitals, you spend this recovery period in the same room in which you delivered. In others, you move to a separate postpartum unit. The nurses continue to monitor your vital signs (blood pressure, pulse, temperature, and breathing) and check the position of your uterus to make sure that it is firm and well contracted. Nurses also monitor your baby's vital signs. Your nurses can provide you with pain medication that your practitioner

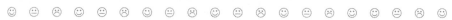
has prescribed, if you need it, and help you care for your episiotomy or cesarean incision, if you have either one.

Bleeding

Vaginal bleeding after delivery is completely normal, even if you had a cesarean delivery. Average blood loss after a vaginal delivery is about 500 cc, or one pint. After a cesarean, average blood loss is twice that — about a liter, or a quart. In order to minimize excessive blood loss, many practitioners give oxytocin (brand name Pitocin) through the mother's intravenous (IV) line or methylergonovine malleate (Methergine) as an intra-muscular injection. These medications help keep the uterus contracted. When the uterus contracts, it squeezes shut the blood vessels from the placental bed to reduce bleeding. If your uterus doesn't seem to be con-tracting well, your doctor or nurse may massage your uterus, through your abdomen, to promote contractions.

The blood coming from your vagina, called *lochia*, may initially appear bright red and contain clots. Over time, it takes on a pinkish and later a brownish color. It gradually diminishes in volume, but the flow may persist for three to six weeks after delivery. You may notice that the amount of bleeding increases each time you breast-feed. This increase happens because the hormones that help produce breast milk also cause your uterus to contract, and this contraction squeezes out any blood or lochia in the uterus. Many patients tell us that the bleeding is heavier when they stand up after being in bed for a while. This extra bleeding happens simply because the blood pools in the uterus and vagina while you're lying down, and when you stand up, gravity draws it out. The best way to deal with postpartum bleeding is to use sanitary napkins. Pads in varying thick-nesses, to accommodate whatever amount of bleeding you have, are avail-able. Tampons are not advised because they may promote infection during the time that your uterus is still recovering.

 If your lochia takes on a foul odor, let your nurse or practitioner know. Also, if you have very heavy bleeding with clots that lasts for several weeks after your delivery, call your practitioner.

Perineal pain

The amount of pain or soreness you feel in your *perineum* (the area between the vagina and the rectum) depends largely on how difficult your delivery was. If your baby came out easily after only a couple of pushes and you have no *episiotomy* (surgical cutting to enlarge the vagina open-ing during labor) or lacerations, you usually feel little pain. But if you pushed for three hours and delivered a 10-pound budding linebacker, you're more likely to have perineal discomfort.

The pain you feel has several causes. First, the baby, as it comes through the birth canal, causes the surrounding tissues to stretch and swell. Also, an episiotomy or tears in the perineum naturally hurt, just as an injury would. The pain is worse during the first two days after delivery. After that, it rapidly improves and is usually nearly gone within a week.

 Many women are concerned about the stitches used to sew up their episiotomy or lacerations. These sutures are not meant to be removed. They gradually dissolve over the next one to two weeks. They are strong enough to handle most activities, so don't worry that a sneeze, a difficult bowel movement, or lifting your 10-pound baby will cause the stitches to tear open.

Swelling

Immediately after delivery, especially after a vaginal delivery, you may discover that your entire body looks swollen. Don't freak out — it's normal. Many women develop swelling during the last few weeks of pregnancy, and this swelling often persists for a few days into the postpartum period. The intense pushing efforts required to deliver the baby may further cause your face and neck to swell, but this also goes away a few days after delivery. In general, it can take up to two weeks for the swelling to completely go away.

 Don't step on the scale the day after you deliver. You may find that you have actually gained weight from all the water you retain during delivery. Your feet may be so swollen that fitting into your normal shoes is difficult. Bring a large, comfortable pair (running shoes or sneakers are good) to wear home from the hospital.

Battle scars

You may find that after delivery, your face is not only swollen but also very red and possibly splotchy. Some women even have black eyes or broken blood vessels around their eyes and, all in all, look as though they've just been in a prize fight. All these characteristics are to be expected; they're caused by the rupture of tiny blood vessels in your face during pushing. Don't be alarmed. You'll look like your old self again in a few days.

Afterpains

The intense contractions that you experienced during labor and delivery that caused your cervix to dilate and helped to push your baby out gradually space out and fade away. But a few persist sporadically after delivery.

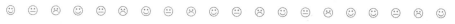

These contractions are called *afterpains* and may be worse or more noticeable while you are breast-feeding. These contractions are completely normal and gradually go away.

Your bladder function postpartum

You may find urinating difficult immediately after delivery, or you may feel discomfort when you do urinate. This discomfort is a result of the way the bladder and urethra are compressed when the baby's head and body come through the vagina. The tissues around the opening to the urethra are often swollen after delivery, and this swelling can add to the discomfort. Some women may need to be catheterized (a thin, flexible plastic tube is inserted through the urethra into the bladder) after delivery to help empty the bladder. Your bladder regains its normal tone a few hours after delivery, so urinary discomfort is usually a short-lived problem.

If you feel primarily a burning sensation during urination, let your doctor or nurse know, because it may be a sign that you're developing a urinary tract infection.

Some women find that they don't have good control over their bladder function. Some women even find that they leak a little urine when they stand up or laugh, or that they have to run like a cheetah to make it to the bathroom in time. If this incontinence happens to you, don't worry too much, because time usually solves the problem. In some cases, it may take a number of weeks to get things under control.

Kegel exercises (see the "Kegel exercises" section later in this chapter) may be useful if the problem persists. Another good strategy is to make a conscious effort to go to the bathroom at regular intervals to empty your bladder before you absolutely have to.

The hemorrhoid blues

Most of your pushing efforts during delivery are focused toward the rectum, a fact that causes many women to develop hemorrhoids — dilated veins that pop out from the rectum. Unfortunately, having no problems with hemorrhoids before you go into labor is no guarantee that they won't appear after delivery. If you develop hemorrhoids during the last part of your pregnancy, they may get worse after delivery. At times, hemorrhoids can be more uncomfortable than an episiotomy, and they last a little longer.

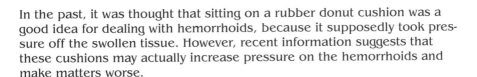

In the past, it was thought that sitting on a rubber donut cushion was a good idea for dealing with hemorrhoids, because it supposedly took pressure off the swollen tissue. However, recent information suggests that these cushions may actually increase pressure on the hemorrhoids and make matters worse.

The good news is that the problem is usually temporary. Postpartum hemorrhoids typically go away within a few weeks. Sometimes, they don't go away completely, but for the most part, they're not bothersome. You may not be troubled by them at all for a few months, they may then be uncomfortable again for a few days, and then they may get better again.

Postpartum bowel function

Many women find that they don't have a bowel movement for a few days after delivery. This lack of bowel function happens for several reasons:

❀ You usually don't eat much food around the time of labor and delivery, so you may have very little waste in your system to get rid of.

❀ Epidurals and some other pain medications sometimes slow down the bowels a little, and your system may take a few days to return to normal.

❀ Many women are afraid of bearing down because they don't want to tear the stitches used to repair their episiotomy, so they avoid having a bowel movement altogether. But doing this is not a great idea. You have no reason to be afraid of tearing the stitches. Your episiotomy is repaired in several layers with strong sutures. Tearing the sutures is extremely difficult, especially by having a bowel movement.

 If you have hemorrhoids or have a laceration that reaches back to the rectal area (see Chapter 9), a bowel movement may be painful. You can reduce the discomfort by using a local anesthetic cream and by using stool softeners. Also, you may want to take a pain reliever shortly before you anticipate having a bowel movement.

Concerning All New Moms

When you're no longer pregnant, your body begins shifting back to its non-pregnancy state, and you're in for a number of changes. This section describes what those changes are, what causes them, and how you can avoid discomfort.

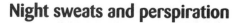

Night sweats and perspiration

If you're managing to get any sleep at night despite having a new baby in the house, you may find that you wake up drenched in sweat. Even during the daytime, you may notice that you perspire significantly more than usual. This sweating is common and is thought to have something to do with fluctuations in hormone levels that occur as your body returns to a non-pregnant state. It is very similar to the night sweats and hot flashes that menopausal women get, due to a drop in estrogen levels. As long as the sweating is not associated with any fever, it's not a problem. It goes away over the course of the next month or so.

Bathing

Traditionally, doctors told women not to take deep tub baths after delivery if they were still bleeding. Today, many practitioners say that tub baths are okay, and most feel that sitz baths (soaking your bottom in a small amount of warm water) are perfectly acceptable. If your practitioner feels that it's better for you to wait until your bleeding has subsided, he or she is concerned that full baths may increase the chance that you develop an infection inside your uterus. The trouble is that doctors really have no data on this topic — no studies demonstrate a risk from taking full baths. You should ask your practitioner what he or she thinks you should do.

Breast engorgement

A woman's breasts typically begin to engorge — fill with milk — three to five days after she delivers her baby. You may be amazed to see how huge your breasts can really be! If you're breast-feeding, your baby lessens the problem for you as he or she gets the hang of nursing, learns to take in more milk, and establishes a pattern of feeding. At the same time, you also get the hang of breast-feeding, and your nipples stop feeling sore, especially when your baby first latches on. (See Chapter 10 for more information about breast-feeding.)

If you're not breast-feeding, you may find that your breasts stay engorged for 24 to 48 hours (which can be quite painful), and then begin to feel better. Wearing a tight-fitting supportive bra may make you more comfortable. Applying ice packs or bags of frozen peas to your breasts helps the milk to "dry up," as does taking cold showers. Cold temperature causes the blood vessels in the breasts to constrict, lessening milk production, while warmth causes the blood vessels to dilate, promoting milk production.

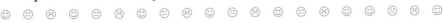
Stretch marks

The majority of women develop some stretch marks during pregnancy. If you don't, you're one of the lucky few. Whether you have them and the extent to which you have them depends in part on how much weight you gain, the type of skin you have, and your basic genetic propensity to develop stretch marks. The marks usually fade over the course of several months after delivery. In light-skinned women, stretch marks become silvery white; in dark-skinned women, they turn lighter brown. Many women apply vitamin E, creams, lotions, and other concoctions to their stretch marks, but these products are generally not effective. While doctors have found no cure for stretch marks, some dermatologists are trained in laser techniques that may reduce the extent of the stretch marks considerably.

Hair loss

One of the stranger aspects of the postpartum return to normalcy is hair loss. A few weeks or months after delivery, most women notice that they're shedding like crazy. This shedding is normal. It is one of the effects that estrogen has on your body during pregnancy. This common problem doesn't last long. Your hair is usually back to normal by nine months after delivery.

Getting Back to Exercise

It typically takes six to eight weeks for the changes that your body experiences during pregnancy to disappear — which means that, after delivery, your body needs some time to get back in shape for vigorous exercise. Resume your sports and workouts gradually. Naturally, the amount of exercise you can handle depends on what kind of shape you were in before and during your pregnancy. Whatever your condition, make exercise a priority. Fitness has many important benefits for both your physical and emotional well-being. It can help your body recover from the stress of pregnancy, and it helps you feel more even-tempered and better about yourself.

Kegel exercises

Kegel exercises are squeezing motions aimed at strengthening the muscles of the pelvic floor that surround the vagina and rectum. These muscles give support to the bladder, rectum, uterus, and vagina. Keeping them strong is key to reducing the adverse effects that pregnancy and delivery can have on this part of the body. If the pelvic floor muscles are very weak, the chances are greater that you will develop urinary stress incontinence — a leakage of urine when you cough, sneeze, laugh, or jump. The chances are also greater that you will have a prolapse or protrusion of the rectum, vagina, and uterus — in which these organs begin to sag below the pelvic floor.

Pregnancy places extra weight on the pelvic floor muscles, and vaginal delivery stretches and puts added pressure on them. The net result is a general weakening. Some women seem to naturally maintain excellent muscle tone in the pelvic floor after delivery. But others notice symptoms of weakness: a little urinary incontinence, the feeling that their vagina is loose, or pressure on their pelvic floor from a sagging uterus, vagina, or rectum. The way to strengthen the pelvic floor muscles — to avoid or diminish these symptoms — is to perform Kegel exercises.

To perform these exercises, you tighten the muscles around your vagina and rectum. Here's a simple way to find out what it feels like to do the exercises correctly: Sometime when you're urinating, try to stop the flow of urine mid-stream. Or insert a finger in your vagina and try to tighten the muscles around your finger. If you're doing Kegels correctly, your finger feels the squeeze. (Both of these techniques are simply ways of figuring out how to squeeze the muscles, not the way you normally practice the exercise.)

When you're first doing Kegels, squeeze the muscles for only a few seconds and then release. Squeeze five to ten times per session, and try to do three to four sessions a day. Ultimately, you can build up to the point where you hold each squeeze for ten seconds and do 25 squeezes per session. You should continue to do the Kegels four times a day. You can do them while you're sitting, standing, or lying down, and you can do them while you're also doing something else — bathing, cooking, talking on the phone, watching television, driving your car, or standing in line at the grocery store.

Abdominal exercises

Over the course of two weeks, depending on how you feel, you can gradually increase your exercising until you're fully active again. Finding the time may be a problem, of course. But fitting exercise into your schedule is worth every effort. Taking care of a newborn can make you feel as though you've just run a marathon, but real exercise is what your body needs. In fact, by improving your overall sense of well-being, exercise can make the whole challenge of caring for a new baby much easier.

The thing you must do to restore strength to your abdominal muscles is contract them. Any number of styles of abdominal exercises called *crunches* work fine.

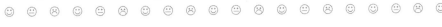
A good abdominal exercise is the most basic, simple one: Lie on your back with your knees bent and feet flat on the floor a few inches apart. Raise your head and shoulders three to six inches above floor level. When you do this exercise correctly, you can literally feel your abdominal muscles tightening. Start with three sets of 8 or 10, and see whether you can work up to doing three sets of 16.

Working your lower abdominals is also important. One good exercise is to lie on the floor with your legs lifted up in the air at about a 90-degree angle. Slowly lift your bottom an inch or two off the floor, breathing out as you do. Try doing 8 to 10 repetitions, rest for a while, and then repeat — and repeat again. After a while, you can work yourself up to doing 15, 20, or even 30 in a row.

 You can also do some exercises with your baby — and get the most out of playtime. Lying on your back, lift your legs up and bend your knees at a 90-degree angle. Then you can lay your baby stomach-down on your lower legs and lift your head and shoulders upward, reaching your face toward your baby's. Start with three sets of 5.

You can also do push-ups while playing with your baby. Just lay the baby on the floor and position your hands on either side, with your body stretched out away from the baby. Start with your arms straight and then slowly bend your elbows to lower your body until you're close enough to touch your nose to your baby's. Straighten your arms to raise your body; repeat. If you're not strong enough to do a standard push-up, keep your knees on the floor. Try to start with two sets of 10 and work your way up to two sets of 15 or 20 (on the toes).

When your baby is old enough to hold up his or her head, you can try the simple — and fairly self-explanatory — baby bench press: Lie flat on your back, hold your baby to your chest, and simply (and gently) lift him or her straight up in the air — again and again. Start with two sets of 10. Later on, try for three sets.

 Walking is great exercise for just about everyone. During the first two weeks after delivery, take it slowly. But after that, you may find that long or brisk walks are enjoyable for you and your baby — and a great form of exercise.

Your Postpartum Diet

Any woman who's just had a baby needs to once again examine her diet. If you're breast-feeding, you want to make sure, as you did when you were pregnant, that you're eating a healthy combination of foods that provide both you and your baby with good nutrition. You also need to make sure you are getting enough fluid. What's more, many women who have just delivered babies are eager to return to their pre-pregnancy weight.

Losing the weight

You may feel like jumping onto a scale right after delivery to see how much weight you've lost. But take caution: Some women do lose a lot of weight quickly after delivery, but some actually gain weight from all the fluid retention. Rest assured that you will soon weigh less than you did before you delivered, probably about 15 pounds less, but the loss may not register until a week or two after delivery.

Here's what accounts for the initial weight loss:

❀ **Baby:** 6 to 9 pounds

❀ **Placenta:** 1 to 2 pounds

❀ **Amniotic fluid:** 1 to 2 pounds

❀ **Maternal fluids:** 4 to 8 pounds

❀ **Shrinking uterus:** 1 pound

Your uterus continues shrinking for several weeks. Immediately after you deliver, it still extends up to about the level of your navel — about the same point as when you were 20 weeks pregnant. However, because of the excess skin you now have, you probably still look pregnant when you stand up. Don't let your appearance get you down! Your uterus keeps contracting, and your skin regains much of its tone until, by about two months after delivery, your belly is down to its pre-pregnancy size.

Most women need two to three months to get back to their normal weight, but, of course, the time varies according to how much weight you gain during pregnancy. If you gain 50 pounds (and had just one baby), don't expect to look fabulous in a bikini six weeks after you deliver. Sometimes, a woman needs an entire year to get back into shape. A healthy diet and regular exercise help the weight come off.

Try to get as close to your pre-pregnancy weight — or your ideal body weight — as soon as is reasonably possible. You don't have to let a pregnancy turn into a permanent weight gain. If you let each successive pregnancy cause a little more accumulation, your health may suffer in the long run.

To help you lose weight, use Table 13-1. Enter your starting weight at Week 1, and then, with each passing week, record what you weigh. With perseverance and a little luck, you can get down to your pre-pregnancy weight.

☺ ☺ ☹ ☺ ☺ ☹ ☺ ☺ ☹ ☺ ☺ ☹ ☺ ☺ ☹ ☺ ☺ ☺ ☺ ☹ ☺

Table 13-1 Tracking Your Weight Loss

Week	Your Weight
1	
2	
3	
4	
5	
6	
7	
8	
9	
10	

Taking your vitamins

Whether or not you breast-feed, continue taking your prenatal vitamins for at least six to eight weeks after you deliver. If you do breast-feed, keep taking vitamins until you stop breast-feeding. If you lost a particularly large amount of blood during your delivery, your practitioner may suggest taking iron supplements to help restore your blood count. Calcium is also very important for any woman, especially if you're breast-feeding, in order to keep your bones strong. A calcium supplement or extra calcium in your diet is a good idea.

Having Sex Again

If you're like most women postpartum, sex is the last thing you want to think about. Many women find that their interest in sex declines considerably during the first weeks and months after pregnancy. But at some point, the fatigue and emotional stress of childbirth ease up, and your thoughts are likely to be more amorous again. For some lucky women, the rebound occurs fairly quickly. For others, it may take 6 to 12 months.

The drastic hormonal shifts that occur after delivery directly affect your sex organs. The precipitous drop in estrogen leads to a loss of lubrication for your vagina, and less engorgement of blood vessels, as well. (Increased blood flow to the vagina is a key aspect of sexual arousal and orgasm.) For these reasons, intercourse after childbirth can be painful and sometimes not all that satisfying. With time, as hormone levels return to their pre-pregnancy norm, the problem tends to correct itself. In the meantime, using petroleum jelly or some other lubricant sold specifically for this purpose helps.

The exhaustion and stress of caring for an infant further reduces the desire for sex in some women. Your attention, and your partner's, too, is likely to be focused more on the baby than on the relationship between the parents. It may help to set aside some time for the two of you to be alone together, to be intimate. This time together need not even include sex — just holding, hugging, and expressing feelings for each other.

Giving your body time to heal

Most doctors recommend that women refrain from intercourse for four to six weeks after the baby is born in order to give the vagina, uterus, and perineum time to heal and the bleeding time to subside. At your six-week follow-up doctor visit, you can ask your practitioner about various methods of birth control.

Choosing a contraception method

Many people believe that breast-feeding prevents a woman from becoming pregnant. But while it is true that breast-feeding usually delays the return of ovulation (and, thus, periods), some women who are nursing do ovulate — and do conceive again. You may not ovulate the entire time that you breast-feed, or you may start again as early as two months after delivery. And if you don't breast-feed, ovulation begins, on the average, ten weeks after delivery, although it has been reported to occur as early as four weeks. If you breast-feed for less than 28 days, your ovulation will return at the same time as it does for non-nursing women. So considering your options for birth control before you have sex again is important.

The Baby Blues

The vast majority of women — as many as 80 percent, studies show — suffer a bout of the blues during the first days and weeks after they deliver. Typically, you begin to feel a little down a few days after the birth, and you may continue to feel vague sadness, uncertainty, disappointment, and emotional discontent for a few weeks. Many women are surprised at the feeling — after all, they've looked forward to motherhood, and they feel sure that they're really thrilled about it.

No one knows for sure why women get the postpartum blues, but a few explanations are plausible. First, the shift in hormone levels that comes after delivery can affect mood. Also, when pregnancy ends, a mother must change her whole focus. After focusing on the birth for so many months, she suddenly finds that the big event is over, and she may feel almost a sense of loss. And face it — parenthood brings tremendous anxiety, especially for a first-time mother. Feeling overwhelmed by all the responsibility and all you need to learn about caring for a baby is not unusual for a woman. Add in the physical discomfort — episiotomy repair, breast tenderness, hemorrhoids, fatigue, and the rest — and you begin to wonder how any new mother can avoid feeling a little blue.

If you find yourself suffering from the baby blues, remember that you're not the first woman to feel this way. The feeling is as normal as pregnancy itself. And take heart: Those who have already grappled with the problem have found a number of ways to ease the blues. Here is a list of some of the best strategies:

- **Lack of sleep compounds the problem of the baby blues.** Everything is worse when you're physically fatigued. The amount of stress that you can handle when you've had your rest is much greater than if you haven't slept enough. So try to get more sleep. If the baby is napping, try to lie down and nod off yourself.

- **Accept other people's offers of help.** In most cases, there's no reason you should have to take care of your baby entirely by yourself. You're a great mom, even if you do let Aunt Suzie or Grandma Melba change a diaper or burp the baby.

- **Talk about how you feel with other mothers, close family members, and friends.** You're likely to find that they felt exactly as you do now. They can empathize with you and offer suggestions for how to cope.

- **If possible, try to get some time to yourself.** Often, new parents are overwhelmed by the realization that their time is no longer their own. Get out of the house for a while, if you can. Take a walk, read, or watch a movie. Often, the blues are exacerbated by the fact that your body is still not back to what it used to be, and now you no longer have the excuse of being pregnant. So pamper yourself with a manicure or pedicure, a trip to the hair salon, or a massage. Have dinner with your husband or with a friend.

Fortunately, postpartum blues tend to fade away rather quickly, usually by about two to four weeks after the birth. If you don't begin to feel better in three or four weeks, let your practitioner know. Between 10 and 15 percent of women go beyond the blues into full-blown *postpartum depression.* Symptoms include severe unhappiness, an inability to enjoy being with the baby (or life in general), lack of interest in caring for the baby, insomnia, weak appetite, inability to function day to day, extreme anxiety or panic attacks, and even thoughts of harming the baby or yourself.

☺ ☻ ☹ ☺ ☻ ☹ ☺ ☻ ☹ ☺ ☻ ☹ ☺ ☻ ☹ ☺ ☺ ☻ ☹ ☺

Ten Myths about Predicting a Baby's Sex

❀ **Ultrasound can *always* determine the baby's sex.**
Sometimes you can't see between the baby's legs, and sometimes the sonographer is wrong.

❀ **The only way to tell the sex in ultrasound is to see the penis.**
A skilled sonographer can see either a penis *or* a labia if the fetus is in an advantageous position.

❀ **If a woman initiates sex, the baby conceived will be a girl.**
How could this possibly make a difference? A related myth: If the woman's on top when the baby is conceived, it's a boy.

❀ **If a pregnant woman gains weight in her face, the baby is a girl.**
Or if a woman gains weight in her butt, the baby is a boy. The baby's sex has no influence on the way the mother stores fat.

❀ **If a pregnant woman's belly is round, the baby is a girl.**
And if it's bullet-shaped, it's a boy. Forget about it.

❀ **If a woman is moody during pregnancy, the baby is a girl.**
This one is based on the old stereotype of a hysterical female.

❀ **If the fetal heart rate is fast, the baby is a girl.**
And if it's slow, it's a boy. Girls' heart rates are slightly faster, but not to the extent that heart rate can be used as a predictor of sex.

❀ **If a locket dangled over a pregnant woman's abdomen swings back and forth, the baby is a boy.**
If it swings in a circle, the baby is a girl. Or is it the opposite?

❀ **If a pregnant woman sits on a cushion of a sofa that has had a spoon (or a fork) placed under it, she's having a girl (boy).**
What? No.

❀ **Pink Drano means the pregnant woman is carrying a girl.**
Pour a tablespoon of Drano into the toilet bowl and urinate. If the water turns pink — you guessed it — you're carrying a girl. If it turns blue, you're carrying a boy. Anyway, the toilet gets cleaned.

Ten Old Wives' Tales

❁ **The old heartburn myth**
If a pregnant women frequently gets heartburn, her baby will be born with a head of hair.

❁ **The you-can't-be-too-careful myth**
If a pregnant woman steps over a rope, she will choke the baby.

❁ **The curse myth**
Anyone who denies a pregnant woman the food that she craves will get a sty in their eye.

❁ **The ugly-stick myth**
If a pregnant woman sees something ugly or horrible, she will have an ugly baby.

❁ **The java myth**
If a baby is born with *café au lait spots* (light-brown birthmarks), the mother drank too much coffee during pregnancy.

❁ **The myth of international cuisine**
Eating spicy food brings on labor. Not true.

❁ **The great sex myth**
Having passionate sex brings on labor (not true, but go ahead and try it).

❁ **The moon-maid myth**
More women go into labor during a full moon. Although many hospital staffs swear on this one, scientific research doesn't bear it out.

❁ **The myth that no good pregnancy books exist**
You're holding one, aren't you?

❁ **The myth that you can't learn anything new about pregnancy**
A well-informed pregnant woman and her partner know enough not to sweat minor discomforts, inaccurate advice from friends and strangers, and old wives' tales.

Index

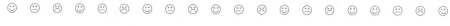

Index

continued

Index

hepatitis, 40, 112, 125
hiccups, fetal, 58
HIV (human immunodeficiency virus), 40, 125
home pregnancy test, 7
homecare
  baby items checklist, 115–116
  bathing, 116–117, 135–136
  burping, 118, 128
  crying, 95–96, 110, 118–120
  massaging your baby, 148–149
  preparing for, 114–115
  sleeping, 62–63, 118, 139–141, 165
hospital
  admission, 79–80
  fetal heart monitoring, 13, 80–81
  ID bracelets, 112
  newborn care, 111–115
  postpartum care, 153–157
  returning home, 114–115
hot tubs and saunas, 17
human chorionic gonadotropin (hCG), 7, 35
human immunodeficiency virus (HIV), 40, 125
hypoglycemia, 24

☺ **I** ☺

ibuprofen (Motrin), 15, 37
ID bracelets, 112
implantation, 32
implantation bleeding, 6, 42–43
incompetent cervix, 54
incontinence, 65, 156
infant seat, 147
infant warmer, 80
insomnia, 62–63
internal pressure transducer (IPT), 81
iron, 21, 37, 163
ischial spines, 60, 61, 78
itching, 63

☺ **J** ☺

jaundice, 114

☺ **K** ☺

Kegel exercises, 156, 159–160
kicking, 68
knee-chest position, 93

☺ **L** ☺

labor. See also anesthesia; contractions; delivery
  inducing, 70, 81–83
  internal exam for, 78
  pain management, 87–89
  post-term, 70
  potential problems, 86–87
  preterm, 70
  prolonged, 94
  real versus false, 77, 78
  signs of, 67, 76
  stages of, 83–87
  when to call your practitioner, 78–79
lacerations or tears, 102. See also episiotomy
lactation
  benefits of, 124
  fluid consumption and, 129
  stopping, 131–132, 158
lanugo, 108
laxatives, caution for, 38
lifestyle changes, 16–18
lightening or dropping, 61, 76
linea nigra, 48
lithotomy position, 93
liver disorder (cholestasis), 82, 97–98
lochia, 154
lung maturity, 46, 67
lying on your back, 23, 58

☺ **M** ☺

macrosomia, 69
mask of pregnancy (chloasma), 48
massaging your baby, 148–149
mastitis (breast infection), 131
maternal serum alpha-fetoprotein (MSAFP), 49

173

☺ ☻ ☹ ☺ ☺ ☹ ☺ ☻ ☹ ☺ ☺ ☹ ☺ ☻ ☹ ☺ ☺ ☻ ☹ ☺

Index

☺ ☺ ☹ ☺ ☺ ☹ ☺ ☺ ☹ ☺ ☺ ☹ ☺ ☺ ☹ ☺ ☺ ☺ ☺ ☹ ☺